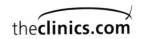

CLINICS IN PERINATOLOGY

Brain Monitoring in the Neonate

GUEST EDITORS
Alan R. Spitzer, MD
Robert D. White, MD

September 2006 • Volume 33 • Number 3

SAUNDERS

An Imprint of Elsevier, Inc.
PHILADELPHIA   LONDON   TORONTO   MONTREAL   SYDNEY   TOKYO

W.B. SAUNDERS COMPANY
A Division of Elsevier Inc.

Elsevier, Inc., 1600 John F. Kennedy Blvd., Suite 1800, Philadelphia, PA 19103-2899

http://www.theclinics.com

CLINICS IN PERINATOLOGY
September 2006
Editor: Carla Holloway

Volume 33, Number 3
ISSN 0095-5108
ISBN 1-4160-3898-1

Reprints. For copies of 100 or more of articles in this publication, please contact the commercial Reprints Department, Elsevier Inc., 360 Park Avenue South, New York, New York 10010-1710. Tel: (212) 633-3813 Fax: (212) 462-1935, e-mail: reprints@elsevier.com.

The ideas and opinions expressed in *Clinics in Perinatology* do not necessarily reflect those of the Publisher. The Publisher does not assume any responsibility for any injury and/or damage to persons or property arising out of or related to any use of the material contained in this periodical. The reader is advised to check the appropriate medical literature and the product information currently provided by the manufacturer of each drug to be administered, to verify the dosage, the method and duration of administration or contraindications. It is the responsibility of the treating physician or other health care professional, relying on independent experience and knowledge of the patient, to determine drug dosages and the best treatment for the patient. Mention of any product in this issue should not be construed as endorsement by the contributors, editors, or the Publisher of the product or manufacturers' claims.

Clinics in Perinatology (ISSN 0095-5108) is published in quarterly by Elsevier Inc., 360 Park Avenue South, New York, NY 10010-1710. Months of issue are March, June, September, and December. Business and Editorial offices: 1600 John F. Kennedy Blvd., Suite 1800, Philadelphia, PA 19103-2899. Customer Service Office: 6277 Sea Harbor Drive, Orlando, FL 32887-4800. Periodicals postage paid at New York, NY and additional mailing offices. Subscription prices are $165.00 per year for (US individuals), $250.00 per year for (US institutions), $195.00 per year (Canadian individuals), $310.00 per year (Canadian institutions), $225.00 per year (foreign individuals), $310.00 per year (foreign institutions) $80.00 per year (US students), and $110.00 per year (foreign students). Foreign air speed delivery is included in all Clinics subscription prices. All prices are subject to change without notice. **POSTMASTER:** Send address changes to *Clinics in Perinatology*; Elsevier Periodicals Customer Service, 6277 Sea Harbor Drive, Orlando, FL 32887-4800. **Customer Service: 1-800-654-2452 (US). From outside of the US, call 1-407-345-1000.** E-mail: hhspcs@harcourt.com

Clinics in Perinatology is also pubilshed in Spanish by McGraw-Hill Interamericana Editores S.A., P.O. Box 5-237, 06500 Mexico D.F., Mexico.

Clinics in Perinatology is covered in *Index Medicus, Current Contents, Excepta Medica, BIOSIS* and *ISI/BIOMED.*

Printed in the United States of America.

GUEST EDITORS

ALAN R. SPITZER, MD, Senior Vice President and Director, The Center for Research and Education, Pediatrix Medical Group, Sunrise, Florida

ROBERT D. WHITE, MD, Director, Regional Newborn Program, Memorial Hospital, South Bend; Clinical Assistant Professor of Pediatrics, Indiana University School of Medicine; Adjunct Professor of Psychology, University of Notre Dame, Notre Dame, Indiana

CONTRIBUTORS

DANA BYRD, PhD, Postdoctoral Fellow, Division of Developmental Psychobiology, Department of Psychiatry, College of Physicians and Surgeons, Columbia University, New York, New York

DONALD CHACE, PhD, Director, Pediatrix Analytical Research Laboratory, Pediatrix Medical Group, Sunrise, Florida

ROBERT R. CLANCY, MD, Professor of Neurology and Pediatrics, University of Pennsylvania School of Medicine; Director, Pediatric Regional Epilepsy Program, The Children's Hospital of Philadelphia, Philadelphia, Pennsylvania

MARIA DELIVORIA-PAPADOPOULOS, MD, Professor of Pediatrics, Department of Pediatrics, Drexel University College of Medicine; Department of Pediatrics, Division of Neonatology, St. Christopher's Hospital for Children, Philadelphia, Pennsylvania

LINDA S. DE VRIES, MD, PhD, Professor in Neonatal Neurology, Department of Neonatology Wilhelmina Children's Hospital, UMC, Utrecht, the Netherlands

ADRÉ J. DU PLESSIS, MBChB, MPH, Director, Neonatal Neurology Research Group, Children's Hospital Boston; Associate Professor, Department of Neurology, Harvard Medical School, Boston, Massachusetts

WILLIAM P. FIFER, PhD, Professor of Psychiatry and Pediatrics, College of Physicians and Surgeons, Columbia University; Assistant Director, Sackler Institute of Developmental Psychobiology, New York State Psychiatric Institute, New York, New York

KAREN I. FRITZ, MD, Associate Professor of Pediatrics, Department of Pediatrics, Drexel University College of Medicine; Department of Pediatrics, Division of Neonatology, St. Christopher's Hospital for Children, Philadelphia, Pennsylvania

STANLEY GRAVEN, MD, Department of Community and Family Health, USF College of Public Health, Tampa, Florida

GORM GREISEN, MD, DMSc, Professor, Department of Neonatology, Rigshospitalet, Copenhagen, Denmark

PHILIP G. GRIEVE, PhD, Assistant Professor of Biomedical Engineering (in Pediatrics), Division of Neonatology, College of Physicians and Surgeons, Columbia University, New York, New York

JILLIAN GROSE-FIFER, PhD, Research Associate, Division of Perinatology, College of Physicians and Surgeons, Columbia University, New York, New York

LENA HELLSTRÖM-WESTAS, MD, PhD, Associate Professor and Senior Consultant, Neonatal Intensive Care Unit, Department of Pediatrics, Lund University Hospital, Lund, Sweden

JOSEPH R. ISLER, PhD, Research Scientist, Division of Neonatolgy, College of Physicians and Surgeons, Columbia University, New York, New York

INGMAR ROSÉN, MD, PhD, Professor of Clinical Neurophysiology, Division of Clinical Neurophysiology, Department of Clinical Science, University Hospital, Lund, Sweden

ALAN R. SPITZER, MD, Senior Vice President and Director, The Center for Research and Education, Pediatrix Medical Group, Sunrise, Florida

MONA C. TOET, MD, PhD, Consultant in Neonatology, Department of Neonatology Wilhelmina Children's Hospital, UMC, Utrecht, the Netherlands

ROBERT D. WHITE, MD, Director, Regional Newborn Program, Memorial Hospital, South Bend; Clinical Assistant Professor of Pediatrics, Indiana University School of Medicine; Adjunct Professor of Psychology, University of Notre Dame, Notre Dame, Indiana

ANDREW WHITELAW, MD, FRCPCH, Professor of Neonatal Medicine, University of Bristol, Bristol, UK

ADAM J. WOLFBERG, MD, MPH, Research Fellow in Neonatal Neurology, Children's Hospital Boston; Department of Neurology, Harvard Medical School; Fellow in Maternal Fetal Medicine, Department of Obstetrics and Gynecology, Tufts New England Medical Center, Boston, Massachusetts

CONTENTS

Preface   xiii
Robert D. White and Alan R. Spitzer

Mechanisms of Injury to the Newborn Brain   573
Karen I. Fritz and Maria Delivoria-Papadopoulos

> Preterm and ill term infants are at risk for brain injury and subse-
> quent neurodevelopmental delay as a result of many perinatal fac-
> tors. Outlined in this article are the basic science mechanisms by
> which hypoxia, hypocapnia, and hypercapnia may result in neuro-
> nal injury in the newborn brain.

**The Physiological Basis for Continuous
Electroencephalogram Monitoring in the Neonate**   593
Ingmar Rosén

> Continuous monitoring of the electrocortical activity as compared
> with intermittent recording sessions offers a possibility of revealing
> changes of the condition of the brain, relevant for clinical decisions.
> Furthermore, trend monitoring, such as amplitude integrated elec-
> troencephalogram (aEEG), helps the clinician in extracting features
> such as background activity, sleep-waking cycling, and seizure pat-
> terns, which have been proven relevant for prognosis and treat-
> ment of the preterm and sick term infant. A coherent model for
> classification and description of neonatal aEEG patterns is pre-
> sented.

Brain Monitoring in the Neonate—the Rationale   613
Gorm Greisen

> Experts argue that no brain monitoring of clinical value is currently
> available for the very preterm baby. Evidence is lacking about all

parts of the therapeutic package: specificity and sensitivity for severe brain compromise, effectiveness of specific intervention, and overall clinical value over and above standard care. However, brain monitoring will probably be most important ultimately for establishing specific causation between modifiable factors and brain dysfunction or damage.

Amplitude Integrated Electroencephalography in the Full-term Newborn

Linda S. de Vries and Mona C. Toet

619

Amplitude-integrated electroencephalography (aEEG) is beginning to play an important role in the care of full-term infants who have neonatal encephalopathy. The three main features an aEEG provides include (1) the background pattern, showing the activity at admission to the neonatal intensive care unit and the rate of recovery during the first 24 to 48 hours after birth; (2) the presence or absence of sleep-wake cycling; and (3) the presence of most electrographic discharges.

Continuous Electroencephalography Monitoring of the Preterm Infant

Lena Hellström-Westas

633

Continuous electroencephalography (EEG) monitoring provides clinically relevant information in preterm infants. Acute changes during development of intraventricular hemorrhage and white matter injury are associated with EEG and amplitude-integrated EEG (aEEG) deterioration. The early EEG background is also correlated with outcome in preterm infants, although other problems associated with prematurity may influence the long-term prognosis. The limitations of EEG monitoring should be well-understood by users and the continuous EEG monitor should be used as a complement to the standard EEG.

Prolonged Electroencephalogram Monitoring for Seizures and Their Treatment

Robert R. Clancy

649

This article reviews the diagnosis of neonatal seizures using routine electroencephalogram (EEG) examinations and long-term EEG monitoring. EEG is considered the gold standard for identifying the presence and quantifying the burden of neonatal seizures. The most common medication used to treat neonatal seizures is phenobarbital, although its efficacy has never been demonstrated by a formal, randomized, placebo-controlled drug trial.

Training Neonatal Staff in Recording and Reporting Continuous Electroencephalography   667

Andrew Whitelaw and Robert D. White

Continuous electroencephalography can contribute useful information to clinical decision-making in neonatal care. Equipment is now
reliable and user-friendly enough that its use can be taught to medical and nursing staff so that a 24-hour capability is achieved. It is
possible to teach neonatologists, in a 1-day course, background
knowledge on EEG and amplitude-integrated EEG (aEEG), recognition of aEEG patterns that have clinical significance, recognition
of seizures using aEEG and "raw" EEG, the essentials of electrode
placement for aEEG, and interpretation of findings in the clinical
context. This must be followed up by background reading, frequent peer-review sessions on EEG recordings, and a reliable system for storing and access, as well as willingness to consult
experienced operators elsewhere.

High-Density Electroencephalogram Monitoring in the Neonate   679

William P. Fifer, Philip G. Grieve, Jillian Grose-Fifer,
Joseph R. Isler, and Dana Byrd

Early diagnosis of neurologic conditions is crucial for successful
early intervention; therefore, minimally invasive diagnostic procedures are invaluable during the neonatal period. The clinical usefulness of one such technique, the electroencephalogram (EEG), is
well documented. However, the advent of high-density recording
systems has extended its application. High-density EEG recording
uses a significantly increased number of recording sites: 128 to 256
electrodes compared with 10 to 30 in standard recording systems.
This report describes the benefits of using more electrode sites
and highlights the use of related procedures for the assessment
of neural integrity across sensory modalities.

Sleep and Brain Development   693

Stanley Graven

Historically, researchers studying the field of sleep have been divided into two main groups. The first group of sleep studies was
based on behaviors and behavioral sleep. The second group of researchers based their studies on electroencephalogram (EEG) patterns and changes. With technologic advancements, a third group
of researchers is studying sleep using active brain-imaging techniques. Most events that are seen on brain imaging correlate with the
EEG pattern, so that they relate to each other in time and state. Unfortunately, behavioral states do not correlate necessarily with the
EEG changes and vary greatly between animal species. This article
focuses on sleep stages and behaviors that are associated with characteristic EEG patterns.

Near-Infrared Spectroscopy in the Fetus and Neonate   707
Adam J. Wolfberg and Adré J. du Plessis

> Near-infrared spectroscopy allows for real-time, noninvasive mea-
> surement of cerebral hemodynamics and oxygenation at the bed-
> side. This article describes animal and clinical research using
> near-infrared spectroscopy to study cerebral hemodynamic func-
> tion in the fetus, neonate, and child.

**Mass Spectrometry in Neonatal Medicine and Clinical
Diagnostics—the Potential Use of Mass Spectrometry in
Neonatal Brian Monitoring**   729
Alan R. Spitzer and Donald Chace

> This article discusses the application of mass spectroscopy, a tech-
> nology that may have great potential for screening neonatal brain
> injury. This approach is anticipated to become increasingly impor-
> tant in neonatal and perinatal research and newborn care during
> the next few years.

Index   745

FORTHCOMING ISSUES

December 2006
Near-Term Pregnancy and the Newborn
Lucky Jain, MD, MBA,
and Tonse N. K. Raju, MD
Guest Editors

March 2007
Surfactant and Mechanical Ventilation
Steven M. Donn, MD,
and Thomas E. Wiswell, MD
Guest Editors

June 2007
Medical Legal Issues in Perinatal Medicine
Isaac Blickstein, MD, Judy Chervenak, MD, JD,
and Frank Chervenak, MD
Guest Editors

RECENT ISSUES

June 2006
Perinatal Causes of Cerebral Palsy
Marcus C. Hermansen, MD
Guest Editor

March 2006
The Science Behind Delivery Room Resuscitation
Jeffrey M. Perlman, MB ChB
Guest Editor

December 2005
Congenital Heart Disease: Impact on the Fetus, Pregnancy, Neonate, and Family
Gil Wernovsky, MD, Stuart Berger, MD,
and S. David Rubenstein, MD
Guest Editors

The Clinics are now available online!

Access your subscription at
www.theclinics.com

ELSEVIER
SAUNDERS

CLINICS IN
PERINATOLOGY

Clin Perinatol 33 (2006) xiii–xiv

Preface

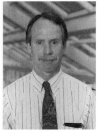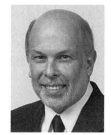

Robert D. White, MD Alan R. Spitzer, MD
Guest Editors

The era of brain monitoring and intervention in perinatal-neonatal medicine is upon us. We have learned a great deal about obstetrical, pulmonary, cardiovascular, and nutritional management of the fetus and newborn, thereby assuring the survival of most of our at-risk patients. Long-term neurologic complications remain common, however, at an unacceptable cost to the child, family and society.

To reduce the incidence and impact of neurologic impairments, we must develop better means of real-time evaluation of brain function, rather than relying on important but chronologically distant follow-up evaluations. In this issue, an international cadre of scientists explores the tools currently available in this fledgling field of brain monitoring in the neonate. Continuous electroencephalogram (EEG) monitoring currently provides the most insight into brain function, so most of this issue is devoted to that modality. After Drs. Fritz and Delivoria-Papadopoulos delineate mechanisms of brain injury in the newborn, Dr. Rosén describes the physiologic basis for continuous EEG monitoring, and Dr. Griesen provides a note of caution before he reviews the rationale for the use of this technology. Brain monitoring in term and preterm infants are presented by Drs. De Vries and Toet, and Dr. Hellström-Westas, respectively.

As in the early stages of many medical advances, access to information often precedes the ability to use it wisely. As the window to the neonatal brain begins to open, the appropriate use of data derived from continuous EEG monitoring is vital, especially with respect to treatment of seizure

doi:10.1016/j.clp.2006.06.007

discharges, for which the article by Dr. Clancy provides guidance. An article by Drs. Whitelaw and White outlining appropriate training and reporting for those using continuous EEG follows, then Dr. Fifer and colleagues complete this section with a glimpse into high-density EEG monitoring, which may provide knowledge that single- or dual-channel EEG monitors cannot.

At every stage in life, sleep is crucial to normal brain function, but it is particularly important in the developing and often healing brain of the newborn. The increasing ability to monitor sleep on a real-time basis is reviewed by Dr. Graven. This issue of *Clinics in Perinatology* then concludes with a look at two more methods of brain monitoring that hold great promise in the near future: near-infrared spectroscopy, reviewed by Drs. Wolfberg and du Plessis, and mass spectrometry, reviewed by Drs. Spitzer and Chace.

We urge the reader to consider these fascinating new technologies and examine their use in the everyday care of the neonate. It is our firm belief that the information provided through brain monitoring will substantially enhance our understanding of neonatal neurologic injury and markedly improve outcomes for all hospitalized newborn infants.

Robert D. White, MD
Regional Newborn Program
Memorial Hospital
615 North Michigan Street
South Bend, IN 46601, USA

E-mail address: Robert_White@pediatrix.com

Alan R. Spitzer, MD
Education, Research and Development
Pediatrix Medical Group
1301 Concord Terrace
Sunrise, FL 33323, USA

E-mail address: Alan_Spitzer@pediatrix.com

ELSEVIER
SAUNDERS

CLINICS IN
PERINATOLOGY

Clin Perinatol 33 (2006) 573–591

Mechanisms of Injury to the Newborn Brain

Karen I. Fritz, MD*,
Maria Delivoria-Papadopoulos, MD

*Department of Pediatrics, Division of Neonatology, St. Christopher's Hospital for Children,
Front and Erie Streets, Philadelphia, PA 19134, USA*

Preterm infants and ill infants are at risk for brain injury, subsequent neurodevelopmental delay, and cerebral palsy caused by hypoxia, ischemia, acidosis, hypoglycemia, and infections, among other insults. Many of these insults may activate similar cell death pathways and lead to necrotic and apoptotic neuronal death. The susceptibility of the newborn brain to damage is determined by various factors, including severity and duration of the event, the presence of antioxidants, membrane lipid composition, and the number and distribution of excitatory N-methyl-D-aspartate (NMDA) receptors.

This article focuses on studies performed in the authors' laboratory using the newborn piglet model and includes known mechanisms of brain injury from hypoxia, hypocapnia, and hypercapnia. Although hyperoxia may lead to brain injury under certain conditions, this topic remains controversial and has been dealt with in a recent issue of *Clinics in Perinatology* [1].

Hypoxia

Hypoxic injury in the fetal and newborn brain results in neonatal morbidity and mortality as well as long-term sequelae, such as mental retardation, seizure disorders, and cerebral palsy [2–4].

Neuronal Ca^{2+} influx

During hypoxia, the hypoxia-induced modification of the NMDA receptor leads to increased intracellular Ca^{2+}, initiating many Ca^{2+}-dependent

Funded by NIH grants HD-20337 and HD-38079.
* Corresponding author.
E-mail address: Karen.Fritz@drexelmed.edu (K.I. Fritz).

pathways of free radical generation, including nitric oxide (NO) [5–7]. Cerebral hypoxia results in increased intracellular Ca^{2+}, which is proportional to the degree of hypoxia [8]. Increased intracellular Ca^{2+} in turn activates proteases, phospholipases, and NO synthase [9,10]. Activation of these enzymes results in the generation of oxygen free radicals, peroxidation of nuclear membrane lipids, and activation of endonucleases leading to fragmentation of nuclear DNA [10–12].

Hypoxia alters nuclear membrane Ca^{2+} influx mechanisms and induces an increase in high-affinity Ca^{2+}-ATPase activity and availability of IP_3 and IP_4 receptor sites, as shown in Figs. 1 and 2 in the guinea pig fetus at term [13]. Hypoxia-induced modification of nuclear membrane Ca^{2+}-influx mechanisms, such as high-affinity Ca^{2+}-ATPase and IP_3 and IP_4 receptors, leads to increased intranuclear Ca^{2+}. The increased intranuclear Ca^{2+} leads to activation of Ca^{2+}/calmodulin kinase (CaM kinase) IV in the nucleus, resulting in phosphorylation of cAMP-response element binding (CREB) protein. In turn, this phosphorylation triggers transcription of apoptotic proteins and fragmentation of nuclear DNA via endonuclease-dependent and caspase-activated DNase (CAD)-mediated mechanisms.

Numerous central nervous system (CNS) processes are controlled by neurotransmitters that act via second messengers (such as Ca^{2+}/calmodulin

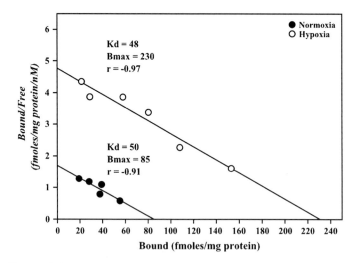

Fig. 1. Characteristics of the IP_3 receptor binding in neuronal cortical nuclei of the guinea-pig fetus at term. ^3H-IP_3 receptor binding was performed in a medium containing 50 mM HEPES (pH 8.0), 2 mM EDTA, ^3H-IP_3 ranging from 7.5 to 100 nM, and 150 μg neuronal nuclear protein. Nonspecific binding was determined in the presence of 10 μM unlabeled IP_3. The K_d and BMax were determined by Scatchard analysis. Representative Scatchard plot for one normoxic (a) and one hypoxic (b) animal is shown. (*From* Zanelli S, Spandou E, Mishra O, et al. Hypoxia modifies nuclear calcium uptake pathways in the cerebral cortex of the guinea-pig fetus. Neuroscience 2005;130:953; with permission.)

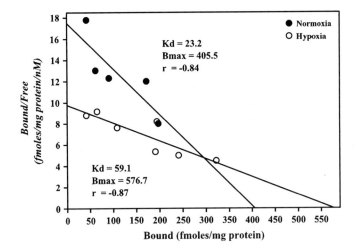

Fig. 2. Characteristics of the IP_4 receptor binding in neuronal cortical nuclei of the guinea-pig fetus at term. ^3H-IP_4 concentrations ranging from 2.5 to 71.5 nM and 150 µg neuronal nuclear protein. Nonspecific binding was determined in the presence of 25 µM unlabeled IP_4. The K_d and Bmax were determined by Scatchard analysis. Representative Scatchard plot for one normoxic (*a*) and one hypoxic (*b*) animal is shown. (*From* Zanelli S, Spandou E, Mishra O, et al. Hypoxia modifies nuclear calcium uptake pathways in the cerebral cortex of the guinea-pig fetus. Neuroscience 2005;130:953; with permission.)

complexes) to modulate the function of key regulatory proteins through phosphorylation and activation of transcription factors that promote gene expression [14]. CaM kinase IV is a member of the CaM kinase cascade that is predominantly localized to the nucleus and mediates Ca^{2+}-regulated gene expression by activating the CREB protein [14,15]. Hypoxia results in an increase in CaM kinase IV activity that is regulated in part by NO [16]. The Ca^{2+} that enters the nucleus enables CaM kinase IV to phosphorylate Ser^{133} of the CREB protein in a process that is a cAMP-independent [17,18]. The binding of CREB to CRE (cAMP-responsive element) does not itself induce transcription unless phosphorylation of CREB at Ser^{133} has occurred [18]. CREB-binding protein (CBP) and p300 are coactivators that interact with the phosphorylated form of CREB and induce transcription of genes containing CRE sequences such as c-fos [18,19]. CREB binding protein connects sequence-specific activators to components of the transcription apparatus [19,20].

The CaM kinase IV-mediated increased phosphorylation of CREB protein triggers transcription of apoptotic proteins, such as Bax and Bad, and initiates early events of caspase-mediated programmed neuronal death. During hypoxia, expression of Bax protein increased more than twofold [21]. There was an inverse correlation between the expression of Bax and tissue ATP and PCr levels [22]. Bcl-2 protein expression did not change significantly during hypoxia. Therefore, the ratio of Bax to Bcl-2 protein increased more than 200% during hypoxia as compared with normoxia.

Induction of apoptosis

Proapoptotic proteins initiate programmed cell death by activating caspases. Caspases are a unique family of proteases that play an important role in the initiation and execution of apoptosis [23,24]. All caspases contain a cysteine residue at their active site and specifically cleave substrate proteins at an aspartic acid residue. There are two main classes of caspases: class I and class II. Class I caspases, such as 8, 9, and 10, initiate apoptosis. Class II caspases, such as 3, 6, and 7, are the executioner caspases and are responsible for the breakdown of cells [25,26].

Hypoxia results in increased activation and expression of caspase-3, caspase-8, and caspase-9 in the cerebral cortex of newborn piglets [27]. Activated caspase-3 cleaves numerous intracellular proteins, such as actin, fodrin, and lamins, which maintain cell structure. It also cleaves and inactivates nuclear enzymes, such as poly (ADP-ribose-polymerase (PARP) and the inhibitor of caspase-activated DNase (ICAD). Inactivation of PARP, which is a DNA repair enzyme, leads to cessation of cellular DNA repair, whereas inactivation of ICAD leads to activation of caspase-activated DNase (CAD), which then cleaves chromosomal DNA. This sequence results in disruption of cell nuclei and the morphologic changes that are characteristic of apoptosis [23,28].

We have shown that nuclear genomic DNA fragmentation correlates with the degree of cerebral tissue hypoxia in newborn piglets [29]. The degree of neuronal cortical genomic DNA fragmentation secondary to hypoxia correlated exponentially with ATP and phosphocreatine concentration [22]. The results of these studies demonstrate that fragmentation of nuclear DNA increases with the increase in cerebral tissue hypoxia.

During hypoxia there is increased generation of oxygen free radicals and lipid peroxidation as measured by conjugated diene production in the cerebral cortex of newborn piglets, demonstrated in Figs. 3 and 4 [30]. These alterations are attenuated by pretreatment with indomethacin, possibly through altering cerebral blood flow during hypoxia.

It is clear that hypoxia results in a series of cellular events that leads to neuronal death. During hypoxia, the NMDA receptor-mediated increase in intracellular Ca^{2+} initiates several reactions, including activation of NO synthase (yielding synthesis of NO), production of free radicals, damage to cellular structural proteins, changes in gene expression, and events leading to cellular death [8,31].

Nitric oxide adversely affects neurons by reacting with superoxide to form peroxynitrite, a toxic free radical that is known to alter cell membranes by increasing the activity of Ca^{2+} ATPase and by increasing intranuclear Ca^{2+} [32]. Administration of NO synthase inhibitors, and thereby NO production, prevented the hypoxia-induced generation of free radicals, nitration of NMDA receptor subunits, calmodulin kinase IV activation, phosphorylation of CREB protein at Ser^{133}, expression of the

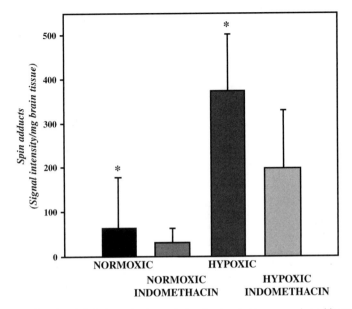

Fig. 3. Spin adduct levels in indomethacin treated and untreated in normoxic and hypoxic new-born piglet cerebral cortices. The data are mean ± SD. (*From* Torres L, Anderson C, Marro P, et al. Cyclooxygenase-mediated generation of free radicals during hypoxia in the cerebral cortex of newborn piglets. Neurochem Res 2004;29:1828; with permission.)

proapoptotic protein Bax, and fragmentation of nuclear DNA (see Refs. [7,33–36]).

To summarize, cerebral tissue hypoxia leads to activation of nuclear Ca^{2+} influx mechanisms, such as the high-affinity Ca^{2+} ATPase, resulting in increased neuronal nuclear Ca^{2+} influx. Increased intranuclear Ca^{2+} increases expression of the proapoptotic gene Bax compared with the antiapoptotic gene Bcl-2. Increased Bax protein activates caspase-9 and caspase-3, which degrade cytoskeletal proteins and lead to the fragmentation of genomic DNA. In addition, the hypoxia-induced increase in intranuclear Ca^{2+} may activate Ca^{2+}-dependent endonucleases and lead to fragmentation of nuclear DNA. These mechanisms may be controlled by NO and may lead to neuronal death.

Hypocapnia

Hypocapnia occurs in ventilated human newborns and children inadvertently during treatment for increased intracranial pressure and persistent pulmonary hypertension in the newborn, or while on extracorporeal membrane oxygenation [37,38]. Preterm infants and ill infants may be especially at risk for brain injury, subsequent neurodevelopmental delay, and cerebral palsy as a result of hypocapnia-induced alterations in cerebral blood flow (CBF) because they may not be able to precisely autoregulate CBF [39].

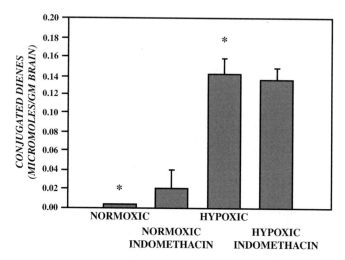

Fig. 4. Levels of conjugated dienes in cerebral cortex of indomethacin treated and untreated normoxic and hypoxic newborn piglets. The data are presented as mean ± SD. (*From* Torres L, Anderson C, Marro P, et al. Cyclooxygenase-mediated generation of free radicals during hypoxia in the cerebral cortex of newborn piglets. Neurochem Res 2004;29:1828; with permission.)

Brain ischemia has been associated with hypocapnia caused by the effect of pH and CO_2 on cerebral vascular tone [40]. In multiple studies, both the degree and duration of hypocapnia have been associated with an increased incidence of PVL and CP in preterm infants [41–43]. However, other studies have not found a relationship between hypocapnia and brain injury [44].

The mechanisms of hypocapnia-induced neuronal injury are unknown. Hypocapnia may alter neuronal nuclear membranes and Ca^{2+} influx through ischemia-induced tissue hypoxia and free radical generation, through alterations in the NMDA receptor, or by increasing the metabolic demands of the neuron [45,46]. Neuronal excitability from hypocapnia is thought to be due to respiratory alkalosis and affects many voltage-gated and ligand channels. An alkalotic pH will increase intrinsic neuronal excitability as well as excitatory or glutamatergic synaptic transmission [47,48]. In addition, respiratory alkalosis has been shown to decrease $GABA_A$-mediated postsynaptic inhibition [49]. Therefore, during hypocapnia, a hyperexcitable state may occur, resulting in increased propensity for seizures and neuronal injury [50].

Alterations in cerebral energy metabolism

In experimental models of newborn hypocapnia, 1 hour of a $PaCO_2$ of 9 to 27 mmHg resulted in a decrease in cortical cerebral energy metabolism in newborn piglets (see Refs. [45,51,52]). In piglets ventilated for 1 hour at a $PaCO_2$ of 9 to 11 mmHg there was an 80% decrease in tissue phosphocreatine (PCr) values; in those ventilated for 1 hour at a $PaCO_2$ of 20 mmHg there was a 38% decrease in tissue PCr levels; and in those ventilated for 1 hour at a $PaCO_2$ of 27 mmHg there was a 13% decrease in PCr levels (see Refs. [45,52,53]). Thus, the degree of reduction of tissue high-energy phosphates correlates with the severity of hypocapnia. The decrease in tissue PCr levels indicates that there was a decrease in tissue oxygenation in the cerebral cortex during hypocapnia.

Hypocapnia may decrease cerebral tissue high-energy phosphates by reducing CBF, thereby decreasing oxygen and nutrient delivery to the brain [40]. In our piglet model, hyperventilation to a $PaCO_2$ of 16 mmHg decreases CBF by 40% [54]. Cerebral oxygenation may be further limited during hypocapnia as alkalosis shifts the oxyhemoglobin dissociation curve to the left and decreases hemoglobin release of oxygen [40]. Brain lactate levels are increased during hypocapnia and are proportional to $PaCO_2$ levels, again suggesting that hypocapnia induces cerebral hypoxia [55]. However, brain lactate production is also tissue pH-dependent, and as pH increases, lactate production increases independent of oxygen availability, so brain and serum lactate levels may reflect tissue oxygenation or tissue pH [56]. The hypocapnic piglets ($PaCO_2$ of 27 mmHg) had an increase in serum lactate levels and heart rate during hypocapnia [52]. These findings may be due to hypocapnia-induced peripheral vasoconstriction. It is also possible that these changes may be due to decreased cardiac output from alterations in the ventilator strategy used. Because arterial blood pressures were constant, however, the increase in ventilator rate used to induce hypocapnia was not thought to decrease cardiac output.

One hour of a $PaCO_2$ of 20 mmHg resulted in an increase in high-affinity Ca^{2+}-ATPase activity (Fig. 5A), increased intranuclear Ca^{2+} influx (Fig. 5B), and nuclear CaM kinase IV activity (Fig. 5C) [51].

Nuclear Ca^{2+} influx

Increased nuclear Ca^{2+} influx is mediated by the high-affinity Ca^{2+}-ATPase enzyme and by inositol 1,4,5-trisphosphate (IP_3) and inositol 1,3,4,5-tetrabisphosphate (IP_4) receptors [57]. Increased intranuclear Ca^{2+} may initiate apoptosis by activating specific enzymes, such as Ca^{2+}/calmodulin-dependent kinase IV (CaM kinase IV), which phosphorylates nuclear proteins and results in the transcription of apoptotic genes [58].

Hypocapnia-induced activation of the nuclear high-affinity Ca^{2+}-ATPase may mediate the increase in intranuclear Ca^{2+} influx seen during hypocapnia. The increase in intranuclear Ca^{2+} may also be mediated by activation of the N-methyl-D-aspartate (NMDA) receptor during hypocapnia. In previous studies, when piglets were ventilated to $PaCO_2$ levels of 9 to 11 mm Hg, there was an increase in spermine and Mg^{++}-dependent activation of the NMDA receptor, presumably allowing an increase in intracellular

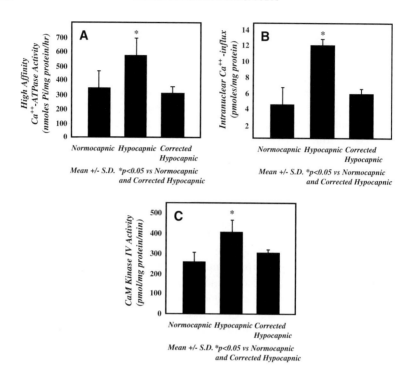

Fig. 5. (*A*) High-affinity Ca^{2+}-ATPase activity in nM Pi/mg protein/h from neuronal nuclei of normocapnic, corrected hypocapnic, and hypocapnic piglets. Data are expressed as a mean ± SD. (*B*) Effect of hypocapnia on neuronal intranuclear Ca^{2+}-influx (pM/mg protein) for normocapnic, corrected hypocapnic, and hypocapnic piglets. Data are mean ± SD. (*C*) Neuronal nuclear CaM kinase activity (pM/mg protein/min) in the cerebral cortex of normocapnic, hypocapnic, and corrected hypocapnic piglets. Data are mean ± SD. (*From* Fritz K, Zubrow A, Ashraf Q, et al. The effects of moderate hypocapnic ventilation on nuclear Ca^{2+}-ATPase activity, nuclear Ca^{2+}flux, and Ca^{2+}/calmodulin kinase IV activity in the cerebral cortex of newborn piglets. Neurochem Res 2004;29(4):794; with permission.)

Ca^{2+} [45]. The increase in intracellular Ca^{2+} activates proteolytic enzymes and results in the generation of oxygen free radicals. Oxygen free radicals may in turn peroxidize nuclear membrane lipids, altering the structure and configuration of the nuclear membrane and its associated proteins. Membrane changes may result in increased intranuclear Ca^{2+} influx and the alteration of nuclear membrane enzymes.

One of the mechanisms of increased intranuclear Ca^{2+} influx is activation of the high-affinity Ca^{2+}-ATPase enzyme. One hour of a $PaCO_2$ of 20 mmHg alters nuclear membrane Ca^{2+} flux mechanisms and specifically activates the nuclear high-affinity Ca^{2+}-ATPase enzyme in the cerebral cortex of newborn piglets. Nuclear calcium signals control a myriad of critical nuclear functions—gene transcription, cell cycle regulation, DNA replication, and nuclear envelope breakdown [50–61]. Therefore, nuclear Ca^{2+} signals are highly regulated. The nuclear envelope, which aids in the regulation of intranuclear Ca^{2+} flux, is made up of an outer and an inner membrane. The outer membrane contains the high-affinity Ca^{2+}-ATPase enzyme and IP_4 receptors, whose activation results in Ca^{2+} accumulation in the perinuclear space [57]. The inner nuclear membrane contains IP_3 receptors, which transport Ca^{2+} into the nucleus from the perinuclear space [62].

Hypocapnia-induced increased intranuclear Ca^{2+} may also result in the activation of Ca-calmodulin-dependent kinases (CaM kinase), such as CaM kinase IV [58]. CaM kinase IV is predominantly located in the nucleus and activates transcription factors, such as cyclic AMP response element binding protein (CREB), by phosphorylating its Ser^{133} site, a necessary step in CREB-mediated transcription [58,63]. Activated CREB then binds to the DNA regulatory sequence cAMP-response element with CREB binding protein and p300, thereby inducing the transcription of apoptotic genes, such as bax, which leads to the activation of capsase-3 and programmed cell death [58,64].

Following both a $PaCO_2$ of 20 and 27 mmHg for 1 hour, CaM kinase IV activity increased in neuronal nuclei of newborn piglets [51,53]. The increase in CaM kinase IV activity during hypocapnia may result in the phosphorylation of CREB and lead to the transcription of apoptotic genes in the cerebral cortex of newborn piglets.

DNA fragmentation

Increased intranuclear calcium activates endonucleases, which cut DNA at intranuclear cleavage sites and results in DNA fragmentation [65]. Unlike control piglets, hypocapnic piglets ($PaCO_2$ 20 or 27 mmHg) displayed a smear pattern of small molecular weight fragments between 100 and 12,000 base-pairs. In piglets with a $PaCO_2$ of 20 mmHg for 1 hour, the density of DNA fragments was eight times higher than in normocapnic controls (Fig. 6). Piglets with a $PaCO_2$ of 27 mmHg also had an increase in DNA fragmentation, with DNA fragment density 2.3 times higher than normocapnic controls [53]. In piglets with a $PaCO_2$ of 27 mmHg for 1 hour, DNA fragmentation varied inversely with levels of ATP and PCr (Fig. 7A and 7B). In the authors' studies, there was a correlation between DNA fragment density and tissue PCr, levels indicating that as tissue oxygenation decreased there was increased fragmentation of nuclear DNA. The linear correlation of PCr and DNA fragmentation did not appear to reflect a direct effect of tissue PCr levels on DNA fragmentation, but rather reflected the trend that as tissue hypoxia worsened, there was an increased fragmentation of DNA. The increase in DNA fragmentation may be due to increased intranuclear Ca^{2+} concentrations, which correlate with tissue PCr values during hypoxia [66].

In both studies, DNA fragmentation occurred after 1 hour of hypocapnia in a smear-type pattern. The time frame and smear pattern suggest that

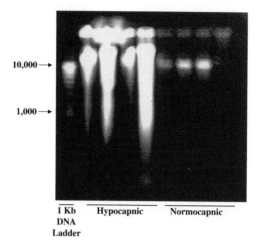

Fig. 6. Gel electrophoresis of cortical DNA fragmentation in hypocapnic (a $PaCO_2$ of 20 mmHg for 1 h) and normocapnic newborn piglets using a standard 1-kb DNA latter. (*From* Fritz K, Ashraf Q, Mishra O, et al. Effect of moderate hypocapnic ventilation on the nuclear DNA fragment and energy metabolism in the cerebral cortex of newborn piglets. Pediatr Res 2001;50:587; with permission.)

fragmentation is due to the activation of proteases and necrotic cell injury rather than programmed cell death. However, the smear pattern of degradation observed in this study may be the result of the action of proteases or the incomplete digestion of DNA by endonucleases. When intranuclear Ca^{2+} increases, nuclear proteases are activated, leading to the digestion of histone proteins. If protease activation precedes the activation of endonucleases, then degradation of histone proteins will allow random access of endonucleases to DNA and result in additional sites for the action of endonucleases and a nonspecific or smear pattern of DNA fragmentation. However, if endonucleases are activated first, before protease activation, they will cleave DNA at specific internucleosomal regions, producing a nucleosome-sized ladder pattern [65]. In this study, as in others, DNA fragmentation is not a hallmark of programmed cell death but indicates that even during a brief episode of moderate hypocapnia there is damage of nuclear DNA and cortical injury in the newborn brain [67].

Piglets ventilated to a $PaCO_2$ of 27 mmHg for 1 hour also had an increase in density of the apoptotic protein Bax compared with normocapnic controls. In these piglets there was no increase in density of the antiapoptotic protein Bcl-2, resulting in an increased ratio of Bax to Bcl-2, a ratio critical to the induction of apoptosis [53].

One hour of either a $PaCO_2$ of 20 or 27 mmHg results in a linear decrease in oxidative metabolism and an increase in intranuclear Ca^{2+} flux that may be due to an increase in activation of the high-affinity CaATPase enzyme. It may also result in activation of the CaM kinase IV enzyme, expression of

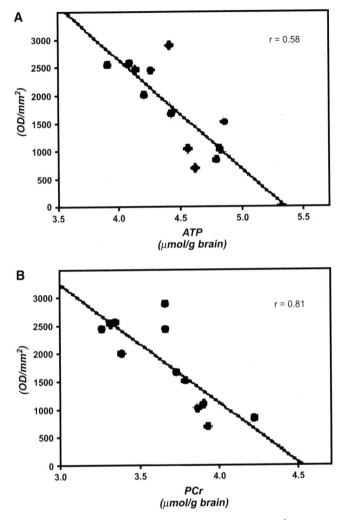

Fig. 7. Linear correlation of nuclear DNA fragment density (OD/mm²) and tissue ATP (*A*); and phosphocreatine (PCr) (*B*) levels in the cerebral cortex of hypocapnic (a PaCO₂ of 27 mmHg for 1 h) and normocapnic piglets, *P* = .01 for graphs A and B. (*From* Fritz K, Zubrow A, Ashraf Q, et al. The effects of hypocapnia (PaCO₂ 27mmHg) on CaM kinase IV activity, Bax/Bcl-2 protein expression and DNA fragmentation in the cerebral cortex of newborn piglets. (Neurosci Lett 2003;352:214; with permission.)

proaptotic proteins, fragmentation of nuclear DNA, and apoptotic neuronal death in the newborn brain.

The authors speculate that hypocapnia-induced tissue hypoxia leads to the generation of free radicals that modify nuclear membrane proteins by lipid peroxidation, resulting in increased nuclear Ca^{2+} influx. The hypocapnia-induced increase in intranuclear Ca^{2+} may result in endonuclease activation, leading to DNA fragmentation in the cerebral cortex of newborn brain and increased CaM kinase activity. The Ca^{2+}-induced increase in CaM kinase IV activity during hypocapnia may also result in the phosphorylation of CREB protein, producing increased transcription of proapoptotic genes in the cerebral cortex of newborn piglets.

Hypercapnia

The long-term neurologic morbidity for preterm newborns and ill newborns remains a serious concern. Among these infants, hypercapnia is a common occurrence. Current clinical practice often allows infants ventilated acutely or chronically to remain hypercapnic (permissive hypercapnia) to limit ventilator-induced lung injury. The effects of hypercapnia on the newborn brain are controversial, as there is not a known safe range of $PaCO_2$.

Recent clinical studies have not shown an immediate harmful effect of hypercapnia in human infants [68–70]. However, in most of these studies, long-term neurologic outcomes were not reported. In addition, subtle alterations in brain structure and function may not be detectable in these clinical studies.

Hypercapnia ($PaCO_2 > 60$ mmHg) results in increased CBF and decreased cerebral vascular resistance in newborn infants [71–73]. It has been associated with intraventricular hemorrhage (IVH) in some studies but not in others [74–78]. There are some clinical data suggesting that hypercapnia may be harmful to the newborn brain even if it does not result in IVH (see Refs. [4,75,76]). Moderate elevations in $PaCO_2$ (end tidal PCO_2 of 60 mmHg) in healthy preterm (33–36 weeks) infants significantly impeded brain stem auditory-evoked responses [79]. In other studies, low-birthweight infants and term infants with impaired cerebral blood flow reactivity during hypercapnia had poor neurologic outcomes or developed hypoxic-ischemic encephalopathy [80,81].

In the authors' studies, the effects of two levels of elevated $PaCO_2$ on the newborn brain, a $PaCO_2$ of 65 mmHg and a $PaCO_2$ of 80 mmHg are described [82]. The data demonstrate a decrease in high-energy phosphates, an increase in CaMK IV activity, an increase in phosphorylation of CREB protein, and increased Bax protein expression in piglets exposed to either a $PaCO_2$ of 65 mmHg or a $PaCO_2$ of 80 mmHg compared with normocapnic piglets. The pH of the animals with a $PaCO_2$ of 80 mmHg (7.25 ± 0.01) was not statistically different than of the animals with a $PaCO_2$ of 65 mmHg (7.30 ± 0.06).

Hypercapnia (either a $PaCO_2$ of 65 mmHg or a $PaCO_2$ of 80 mmHg) resulted in an increase in nuclear CaM K IV activity. The increase in CaM K IV activity seen during hypercapnia may be due to hypercapnia-induced intracellular acidosis [82]. The isoelectric point of CaM K IV is 4.65, indicating that the enzyme will be fully charged in an acidotic environment.

Activity of CaM K IV is increased during acidosis [83,84]. In the carboxy region of the molecule, there is a stretch of amino acids, of which 81% are glutamate residues, including a string of 11 glutamate residues [85]. During hypercapnia-induced acidosis, these glutamate residues may be fully ionized, allowing maximal enzyme activity.

During both levels of hypercapnia there was an increase in phosphorylated CREB Ser[133] protein density in the cerebral cortex of newborn piglets compared with normocapnic piglets, as shown in Fig. 8. Activation of the cerebral NMDA receptor results in increased intracellular Ca^{2+}, which may potentiate Ca^{2+} flux into the nucleus and increase CaM K IV activity and CREB phosphorylation. Increased CREB Ser[133] phosphorylation depends on intranuclear Ca^{2+} concentrations and intracerebroventricular injection of NMDA potentiates binding of CREB protein to DNA in mice [86]. In addition, both the phosphorylation and the activity of CaM K IV are increased by increasing intracellular Ca^{2+} flux through glutamate-induced NMDA receptor activation [87]. Hypercapnia-induced acidosis may result in alteration of the NMDA receptor and increase NMDA receptor-mediated intracellular Ca^{2+} influx, resulting in an increase in nuclear Ca^{2+} influx, phosphorylation of CREB protein, and gene transcription in newborn piglets.

When CREB protein is phosphorylated, there is an increase in the spherical site and net positive surface charge of the CREB/DNA complex. Therefore, it appears that phosphorylation of CREB protein alters its binding affinity, its secondary structure, and the charge characteristics of the molecule, all of which may be enhanced in an acidotic environment [88].

During hypercapnia there was an increase in expression of Bax protein, resulting in an increased ratio of the proapoptotic protein Bax to the anti-apoptotic protein Bcl-2, compared with normocapnic piglets as shown in Fig. 9. During hypercapnia, the increase in Bax protein and ratio of Bax/Bcl-2 indicates a propensity of the cells to undergo programmed cell death in the newborn piglet brain.

In addition to Bax, hypercapnia has been shown to induce the expression of other nuclear proteins as well. The nuclear protein FOS is expressed in

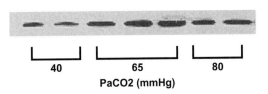

Fig. 8. Representative Western blots of phosphorylated CREB Ser[133] protein expression in pCO$_2$ 40, pCO$_2$ 65, and pCO$_2$ 80 groups in neuronal nuclei of newborn piglets. The bands were visualized at a molecular weight of 43 kD. (*From* Fritz KI, Zubrow AB, Mishra OP, et al. Hypercapnia-induced modifications of neuronal function in the cerebral cortex of newborn piglets. Pediatr Res 2005;57:301; with permission.)

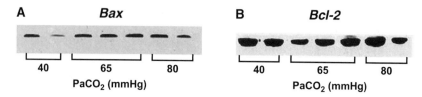

Fig. 9. Representative Western blots of Bax (*A*) and Bcl-2 (*B*) protein expression in neuronal nuclei of newborn piglets from the pCO_2 40, pCO_2 65, and pCO_2 80 groups. (*From* Fritz KI, Zubrow AB, Mishra OP, et al. Hypercapnia-induced modifications of neuronal function in the cerebral cortex of newborn piglets. Pediatr Res 2005;57:301; with permission.)

brainstem chemosensitive neurons during hypercapnia [89]. FOS expression appears to be mediated by activation of MAP kinases, PKC_α, and PKC_β [90]. Therefore, it appears that hypercapnia leads to the activation of kinases and the subsequent expression of neuronal apoptotic proteins.

During hypercapnia, neuronal injury may result from alterations in CBF, decreased extracellular and intracellular pH, the generation of oxygen free radicals, or increased intracellular and intranuclear Ca^{2+} flux.

It is possible that during hypercapnia the ensuing respiratory acidosis alters brain cell membranes and results in increased CaM K IV activity, phosphorylation of CREB protein, and Bax protein expression in the cerebral cortex of newborn piglets.

During hypercapnia, there is a decrease in extracellular (pH_e) and intracellular (pH_i) pH [91–93]. The hypercapnia-induced intracellular acidosis has been shown to retard oxidative phosphorylation. Nuclear magnetic resonance studies during hypercapnia demonstrated that there was a linear correlation between Pi/NTP and brain pH_i [92]. During hypercapnia ($PaCO_2$ 98 ± 3 mmHg) in newborn lambs there was a significant increase in the ratio of Pi to nucleotide triphosphates and a significant decrease in the ratio of PCr to Pi. The impact of hypercapnia on cellular metabolism with the hypercapnia-induced decrease in high-energy phosphates is demonstrated here. The decrease in tissue levels of ATP and PCr in the newborn piglets in this study was assumed to be the result of increased metabolic demand on the neurons to maintain ionic homeostasis during acidosis.

In tissue slices and cultured astrocytes, a reduction in pH_e leads to brain edema and cell necrosis [94–96]. During hypercapnia, when pH_i and pH_e are lowered, restitution of normal pH_i may not be feasible, resulting in neuronal injury and possibly cell death through activation of nuclear transcription mechanisms. It has been suggested that the hypercapnia-induced increase in intracellular [H^+] may compete for binding sites with intracellular Ca^{2+}, resulting in an increase in free cytosolic Ca^{2+} [97]. The authors propose that a hypercapnia-induced increase in intracytosolic Ca^{2+} results in an increase in intranuclear Ca^{2+} influx, as membrane enzymes are altered by acidosis. The increase in intranuclear Ca^{2+} then may activate CaM K

IV, phosphorylation of CREB, and the transcription of apoptotic genes, as demonstrated in this current study.

The two groups of piglets, the pCO_2 65 and pCO_2 80 groups, had a similar decrease in high-energy phosphates, increased CaM K IV activity, increased phosphorylation of CREB protein, and increased expression of Bax protein. However, even though these groups had statistically different levels of $PaCO_2$, the pH range for each group was not statistically different. The effects of hypercapnia on the brain are likely due to decreases in pH and not differences in $PaCO_2$.

Summary

The authors conclude that 6 hours of either a $PaCO_2$ of 65 mmHg or 80 mmHg alters nuclear enzyme activity and protein expression in the cerebral cortex of newborn piglets. Specifically, hypercapnia results in a decrease in cerebral energy metabolism, an increase in CaMK IV activity, phosphorylation of CREB protein, and the expression of apoptotic proteins. The acidosis induced by hypercapnia may be deleterious to the newborn brain and alter nuclear membrane enzymes, producing an increase in intranuclear Ca^{2+} that results in an increase in CaMK IV activity, the subsequent expression of apoptotic genes, and cell death in the cerebral cortex of the newborn piglet.

References

[1] Richmond S, Goldsmith J. Air or 100% oxygen in neonatal resuscitation? Clin Perinatol 2006;33:11–27.

[2] Raichle M. The patholophysiology of brain ischemia. Ann Neurol 1983;13:2–10.

[3] Vannucci R. Experimental biology of cerebral hypoxia-ischemia: relation to perinatal brain damage. Pediatr Res 1990;27:317–26.

[4] Volpe J. Neurology of the newborn. 3rd ed. Philadelphia: WB Saunders; 2000.

[5] Mishra O, Fritz K, Delivoria-Papadopoulos M. NMDA receptor and neonatal hypoxic brain injury. Ment Retard Dev Disabil Res Rev 2001;7:249–53.

[6] Mishra O, Zanelli S, Ohnishi S, et al. Hypoxia-induced generation of nitric oxide free radicals in cerebral cortex of newborn guinea pigs. Neurochem Res 2000;25:1559–65.

[7] Numagami Y, Zubrow A, Mishra O, et al. Lipid free radical generation and brain cell membrane alteration following nitric oxide synthase inhibition during cerebral hypoxia in the newborn piglet. J Neurochem 1997;69:1542–7.

[8] Zanelli S, Numagami Y, McGowan J, et al. NMDA receptor mediated calcium influx in cerebral cortical snyaptosomes of the hypoxic guinea pig fetus. Neurochem Res 1999;24: 437–46.

[9] Halliwel B. Antioxidant defense mechanisms: from the beginning to the end (of the beginning). Free Radic Res 1999;31:261–72.

[10] Mishra O, Delivoria-Papadopoulos M. Cellular mechanisms of hypoxic injury in the developing brain. Brain Res Bull 1999;48:233–8.

[11] Maulik D, Qayyum I, Powell S, et al. Post-hypoxic magnesium decreases nuclear oxidative damage in the fetal guinea pig brain. Brain Res 2001;890:130–6.

[12] Numagami Y, Zubrow A, Mishra O, et al. Lipid free radical generation and brain cell membrane alteration following nitric oxide snythase inhibition during cerebral hypoxic in the newborn piglet. J Neurochem 1997;69:1542–7.

[13] Zanelli S, Spandou E, Mishra O, et al. Hypoxia modifies nuclear calcium uptake pathways in the cerebral cortex of the guinea-pig fetus. Neuroscience 2005;130:949–55.

[14] Hardingham G, Chawla S, Johnson C, et al. Distinct functions of nuclear and cytoplasmic calcium in the control of gene expression. Nature 1997;385:260–5.

[15] Jensen K, Ohmstede C, Fisher R, et al. Nuclear and axonal localization of Ca^{2+}/calmodulin-dependent protein kinase type Gr in rat cerebellar cortex. Proc Natl Acad Sci U S A 1991;88: 2850–3.

[16] Zubrow A, Delivoria-Papadopoulos M, Fritz K, et al. Effect of neuronal nitric oxide synthase inhibition on Ca^{2+}/calmodulin kinase kinase and Ca^{2+}/calmodulin kinase IV activity during hypoxia in cortical nuclei of newborn piglets. Neuroscience 2004;125:937–45.

[17] Ginty D, Kornhauser J, Thompson M, et al. Regulation of CREB phosphorylation in the suprachiasmatic nucleus by light and a circadian clock. Science 1993;260:238–41.

[18] Sheng M, McFadden G, Greenberg M. Membrane depolarization and calcium induce c-fos transcription via phosphorylation of transcription factor CREB. Neuron 1990;4:571–82.

[19] Kwok R, Lundblad J, Chrivia J, et al. Nuclear protein CBP is a coactivator for the transcription factor CREB. Nature 1994;370:223–6.

[20] Kee B, Arias J, Montminy M. Adaptor-mediated recruitment of RNA polymerase II to a signal-dependent activator. J Biol Chem 1996;271:2373–5.

[21] Ravishankar S, Ashraf Q, Fritz K, et al. Expression of Bax and Bcl-2 proteins during hypoxia in cerebral cortical neuronal nuclei of newborn piglets: effect of administration of magnesium sulfate. Brain Res 2001;901:23–9.

[22] Delivoria-Papadopoulos M, Mishra O. Nuclear mechanisms of hypoxic cerebral injury in the newborn. Clin Perinatol 2004;31:91–105.

[23] Nicholson D, Thornberry N. Caspases: killer proteases. Trends Biochem Sci 1997;22: 229–306.

[24] Henkart A. ICE family proteases: mediators of all apoptotic cell death? Immunity 1996;4: 195–201.

[25] Enari M, Talanian R, Wong W, et al. Sequential activation of ICE-like and CPP32-like proteases during Fas-mediated apoptosis. Nature 1996;380:723–6.

[26] Scaffidi C, Fulda S, Srivnivasan A, et al. Two CD95 (APO-1/fas) signaling pathways. EMBO J 1998;17:1675–87.

[27] Khurana P, Ashraf Q, Mishra O, et al. Effect of hypoxia on caspase-3,-8 and -9 activity and expression in the cerebral cortex of newborn piglets. Neurochem Res 2002;27:931–8.

[28] Mukae N, Enari M, Shahira H, et al. Molecular cloning and characterization of human caspase-activated Dnase. Proc Natl Acad Sci U S A 1998;95:9123–8.

[29] Waseem W, Ashraf Q, Zanelli S, et al. Effect of graded hypoxia on cerebral cortical genomic DNA fragmentation in newborn piglets. Biol Neonate 2001;79:187–93.

[30] Torres L, Anderson C, Marro P, et al. Cyclooxygenase-mediated generation of free radicals during hypoxia in the cerebral cortex of newborn piglets. Neurochem Res 2004;29(10): 1825–30.

[31] Christopherson K, Bredt D. Nitric oxide in excitable tissues: physiologic roles and disease. J Clin Invest 1997;100:2424–9.

[32] Gavini G, Zanelli S, Ashraf Q, et al. Effect of nitric oxide synthase inhibition on high affinity Ca^{2+}-ATPase during hypoxia in cerebral cortical neuronal nuclei of newborn piglets. Brain Res 2000;887:385–90.

[33] Zanelli S, Ashraf Q. Mishra, et al. Nitration is a mechanism of regulations of the NMDA receptor function during hypoxia. Neuroscience 2002;112:869–77.

[34] Zubrow A, Delivoria-Papadopoulos M, Ashraf Q, et al. Nitric oxide-mediated $Ca^{+\,+}$/calmodulin-dependent protein kinase IV activity during hypoxia in neuronal nuclei from newborn piglets. Brain Res 2002;335:5–8.

[35] Zubrow A, Delivoria-Papadopoulos M, Ashraf Q, et al. Nitric oxide-mediated expression of Bax protein and DNA fragmentation during hypoxia in neuronal nuclei from newborn piglets. Brain Res 2002;954:60–7.

[36] Mishra O, Ashraf Q, Delivoria-Papadopoulos M. Phosphorylation of cAMP response element binding (CREB) protein during hypoxia in cerebral cortex of newborn piglets and the effect of nitric oxide synthase inhibition. Neuroscience 2002;115:985–91.

[37] Laffey J, Kavanagh B. Hypocapnia. New Engl J Med 2002;347:43–53.

[38] Graziani L, Gringlas M, Baumgart S. Cerebrovascular complications and neurodevelopmental sequelae of neonatal ECMO. Clin Perinatol 1997;24:655–75.

[39] Volpe J. Neurologic outcome of prematurity. Arch Neurol 1998;55:297–300.

[40] Brian J. Carbon dioxide and the cerebral circulation. Anesthesiology 1998;88:1365–86.

[41] Ikonen R, Janas M, Koivikko M. Hyperbilirubinemia, hypocarbia and periventricular leukomalacia in preterm infants: relationship to cerebral palsy. Acta Paediatr 1992;81:802–7.

[42] Gannon C, Wisweel T, Spitzer A. Volutrama, Paco2 levels, and neurodevelopmental sequelae following assisted ventilation. Clin Perinatol 1998;25:159–75.

[43] Graziani L, Spitzer A, Mitchell D, et al. Mechanical ventilazation in preterm infants: neurosonographic and developmental studies. Pediatrics 1992;90:515–22.

[44] Wiswell T, Granziani L, Komhauser M, et al. High- frequency ventilation in the early management of respiratory distress syndrome is associated with greater risk for adverse outcomes. Pediatrics 1996;98:1035–43.

[45] Graham E, Apostolou M, Mishra O, et al. Modification of the N-methyl D-aspartate (NMDA) receptor in the brain of newborn piglets following hyperventilation induced ischemia. Neuroscience 1996;218:29–32.

[46] Huttunen J, Heinonen E. Effects of voluntary hyperventilation on cortical sensory responses: electroencephalographic and magneto encephalographic studies. Exp Brain Res 1999;125:248–54.

[47] Lee J, Taira T, Pihlaja P, et al. Effects of CO2 on excitatory transmission apparently caused by changes in intracellular pH in the rat hippocampal slice. Brain Res 1996;706:210–6.

[48] Somjen G, Tombaugh G. pH modulation of neuronal excitability and central nervous system functions. In: Kaila K, Ransom BR, editors. pH and brain function. New York: Wiley-Liss; 1998. p. 373–93.

[49] Kaila K. Ionic basis of GABA-A receptor channel function in the nervous system. Prog Neurobiol 1994;42:489–537.

[50] Neidermeyer E, Lopes da Silva F. Electroencephalography: basic principles, clinical applications and related fields. New York: Williams & Wilkins; 1993.

[51] Fritz K, Zubrow A, Ashraf Q, et al. The effects of moderate hypocapnic ventilation on nuclear Ca^{2+}-ATPase activity, nuclear Ca^{2+} flux, and Ca^{2+}/calmodulin kinase IV activity in the cerebral cortex of newborn piglets. Neurochem Res 2004;29(4):791–6.

[52] Fritz K, Ashraf Q, Mishra O, et al. Effect of moderate hypocapnic ventilation on the nuclear DNA fragment and energy metabolism in the cerebral cortex of newborn piglets. Pediatr Res 2001;50(5):586–9.

[53] Fritz K, Zubrow A, Ashraf Q, et al. The effects of hypocapnia ($PaCO_2$ 27mmHg) on CaM kinase IV activity, Bax/Bcl-2 protein expression and DNA fragmentation in the cerebral cortex of newborn piglets. Neurosci Lett 2003;352:211–5.

[54] Hansen N, Nowicki P, Miller R, et al. Alterations in cerebral blood flow and oxygen consumption during prolonged hypocarbia. Pediatr Res 1986;20:147–50.

[55] Van Rijen PC, Luyten PR, van der Sprenkel JW, et al. 1H and 31P NMR measurement of cerebral lactate, high-energy phosphate levels, and pH in humans during voluntary hypoventilation: associated EEG, capnographic and Doppler findings. Magn Reson Med 1989;10:182–93.

[56] Carlisson C, Nilsson L, Siesjo B. Cerebral metabolic changes in arterial hypocapnia of short duration. Acta Anaesthesiol Scand 1974;18:104–13.

[57] Gerasimenko O, Gerasimenko J, Tepikin A, et al. Calcium transport pathways in the nucleus. Eur J Physiol 1996;432:1–6.

[58] Soderling T. The Ca^{2+} calmodulin dependent protein kinase cascade. Trends Biol Sci 1999; 24:232–6.

[59] Karin M. Signal transduction from cell surface to nucleus in development and disease. FASEB J 1992;6:2581–90.

[60] Tombes R, Simerly C, Borisy G, et al. Miosis, egg activation and nuclear envelope breakdown are differentially reliant on Ca^{++} whereas germinal vesicle breakdown is Ca^{++}-independent in the mouse oocyte. J Cell Biol 1992;117:799–811.

[61] Santella L, Carafoli E. Calcium signaling in the cell nucleus. FASEB J 1997;11:1091–109.

[62] Humbert J, Matter N, Artauh J, et al. Inositol 1, 4,5- trisposphate receptor is located to inner nuclear membrane indicating regulation of nuclear calcium signaling by inositol. J Biol Chem 1996;271:478–85.

[63] Hardingham G, Cruzzaleguiu F, Bading H. Mechanisms controlling gene expression by nuclear calcium signals. Cell Calcium 1998;23:131–4.

[64] Chrivia J, Kwok R, Lamb N, et al. Phosphorylated CREB binds specifically to the nuclear protein CBP. Nature 1993;365:855–9.

[65] Tominaga T, Kure S, Narisawa K, et al. Endonuclease activation following focal ischemic injury in the rat brain. Brain Res 1993;608:21–6.

[66] Akhter W, Zanelli S, Ballestero J, et al. Effect of graded hypoxia on neuronal intranuclear calcium influx in newborn piglets [abstract]. Pediatr Res 2000;47:384A.

[67] Collins R, Harmon B, Gibe G, et al. Internucleosomal DNA cleavage should not be the sole criterion for identifying apoptosis. Int J Radiat Biol 1992;61:451–3.

[68] Woodgate P, Davies M. Permissive hypercapnia for the prevention of morbidity and mortality in mechanically ventilated newborn infants. Cochrane Database Syst Rev 2001;(2) CD002061.

[69] Varughese M, Patole S, Shama A, et al. Permissive hypercapnia in neonates: the case of the good, the bad, and the ugly. Pediatr Pulmonol 2002;33:56–64.

[70] Mariani G, Cifuentes J, Carlo W. Randomized trial of permissive hypercapnia in preterm infants. Pediatrics 1999;104:1082–8.

[71] Wyatt J, Edwards M, Delpy D, et al. Response of cerebral blood volume to changes in arterial carbon dioxide tension in preterm and term infants. Pediatr Res 1991;29:553–7.

[72] Leahy F, Cates D, MacCallum M, et al. Effect of CO2 and 100% O2 on cerebral blood flow in preterm infants. J Appl Physiol 1980;48:468–72.

[73] van Bel F, van de Bor M, Baan J, et al. The influence of abnormal blood gases on cerebral blood flow velocity in the preterm newborn. Neuropediatrics 1988;19:27–32.

[74] Wallin L, Rosenfeld C, Laptook A, et al. Neonatal intracranial hemorrhage: II. Risk factor analysis in an inborn population. Early Hum Dev 1990;23:129–37.

[75] Ment L, Oh W, Philip A, et al. Risk factors for early intraventricular hemorrhage in low birth weight infants. J Pediatr 1992;121:776–83.

[76] Szymonowicz W, Yu V, Wilson F. Antecedents of periventricular haemorrhage in infants weighing 1250 g or less at birth. Arch Dis Child 1984;59:13–7.

[77] Levene M, Fawer C, Lamont R. Risk factors in the development of intraventricular haemorrhage in the preterm neonate. Arch Dis Child 1982;57:410–7.

[78] Skouteli H, Kuban K, Leviton A, et al. Arterial blood gas derangements associated with death and intracranial hemorrhage in premature babies. J Perinatol 1988;8:336–41.

[79] Friss H, Wavrek D, Martin W, et al. Brain-stem auditory evoked responses to hypercarbia in preterm infants. Electroencephalogr Clin Neurophysiol 1994;90:331–6.

[80] Muller A, Morales C, Briner J, et al. Loss of C02 reactivity of cerebral blood flow is associated with severe brain damage in mechanically ventilated very low birth weight infants. Eur J Paediatr Neurol 1997;1:157–63.

[81] Pryds O, Greisen G, Lou H, et al. Vasoparalysis associated with brain damage in asphyxiated term infants. J Pediatr 1990;117:119–25.

[82] Fritz KI, Zubrow AB, Mishra OP, et al. Hypercapnia-induced modifications of neuronal function in the cerebral cortex of newborn piglets. Pediatr Res 2005;57:299–304.

[83] Jones D, Glod J, Wilson-Shaw D, et al. cDNA sequence and differential expression of the mouse Ca^{2+}/calmodulin-dependent protein kinase IV gene. FEBS Lett 1991;289:105–9.

[84] Miyano O, Kameshita I, Fujisawa H. Purification and characterization of a brain-specific multifunctional calmodulin-dependent protein kinase from rat cerebellum. J Biol Chem 1992;267:1198–203.

[85] Ohmstede C, Jensen K, Sahyoun N. Ca^{2+}/calmodulin-dependent protein kinase enriched in cerebellar granule cells. Identification of a novel neuronal calmodulin-dependent protein kinase. J Biol Chem 1989;264:5866–75.

[86] Ogita K, Yoneda Y. Selective potentiation of DNA binding activities of both activator protein 1 and cyclic AMP response element binding protein through in vivo activation of N-methyl-D-aspartate receptor complex in mouse brain. J Neurochem 1994;63:525–34.

[87] Kasahara J, Fukunaga K, Miyamoto E. Activation of $CA(^{2+})$/calmodulin-dependent protein kinase IV in cultured rat hippocampal neurons. J Neurosci Res 2000;59:594–600.

[88] Bullock B, Habener J. Phosphorylation of the cAMP response element binding protein CREB by cAMP-dependent protein kinase A and glycogen synthase kinase-3 alters DNA-binding affinity, conformation, and increases net charge. Biochemistry 1998;37:3795–809.

[89] Haxhiu M, Yung K, Erokwu B, et al. CO2-induced c-fos expression in the CNS catecholaminergic neurons. Respir Physiol 1996;105:35–45.

[90] Kuo N, Agani F, Haxhiu M. A possible role for protein kinase C in CO2/H+-induced c-fos mRNA expression in PC12 cells. Respir Physiol 1998;111:127–35.

[91] Wagerle L, Mishra O. Mechanism of CO2 response in cerebral arteries of the newborn pig: role of phospholipase, cyclooxygenase, and lipoxygenase pathways. Circ Res 1988;62: 1019–26.

[92] Cady E, Chu A, Costello A, et al. Brain intracellular pH and metabolism during hypercapnia and hypocapnia in the new-born lamb. J Physiol 1987;382:1–14.

[93] Rosenberg A, Jones M Jr, Traystman R. Response of cerebral blood flow to changes in PCO2 in fetal, newborn, and adult sheep. Am J Physiol 1982;242:H862–6.

[94] Patel K, Hartmann J, Cohen M. Effect of pH on metabolism and ultrastructure of guinea pig cerebral cortex slices. Stroke 1973;4:221–31.

[95] Goldman S, Pulsinelli W, Clarke W, et al. The effects of extracellular acidosis on neurons and glia in vitro. J Cereb Blood Flow Metab 1989;9:471–7.

[96] MacGregor D, Chesler M, Rice M. HEPES prevents edema in rat brain slices. Neurosci Lett 2001;303:141–4.

[97] Siesjo B, Katsura K, Mellergard P, et al. Acidosis-related brain damage. Prog Brain Res 1993;96:23–48.

CLINICS IN
PERINATOLOGY

Clin Perinatol 33 (2006) 593–611

The Physiological Basis for Continuous Electroencephalogram Monitoring in the Neonate

Ingmar Rosén, MD, PhD

*Division of Clinical Neurophysiology, Department of Clinical Science,
University Hospital, S-22185, Lund, Sweden*

The overall aims in the care of the sick newborn are the preservation of brain function and optimal neurologic and developmental outcome. Paradoxically, online continuous functional monitoring in the neonate has traditionally focused on cardiorespiratory variables rather than cerebral function. Electrophysiological brain activity, as reflected by electroencephalogram (EEG), is well established as a tool for providing information about the current functional and metabolic state of the brain and the occurrence of epileptic seizure episodes. In neonatal care, EEG has been used extensively for estimation of the degree of cerebral maturation in preterm infants and for detection of abnormal patterns indicating focal and global cerebral lesions [1–3]. In the neonatal setting, as well as in intensive care in general, the EEG has been recorded intermittently, at best serially rather than continuously. Performing a full multichannel EEG in a newborn requires specialized technical skill in securing correct electrode positioning and impedances, as well as identification of extracerebral biologic and nonbiologic artifact sources. Interpretation of neonatal EEG is considered among clinical neurophysiologists a demanding task that must consider the specific EEG features related to different gestational age, activity state, and medication.

The main disadvantage with intermittent conventional EEG during neonatal care is the difficulty in discriminating emerging trends of development of the electrocerebral activity over hours and days. If possible at all, it takes special skills not usually available in the neonatal intensive care unit (NICU) to identify long-term changes of EEG patterns. To have an impact on

This work has been supported by grant 84 from the Swedish Research Council.
E-mail address: ingmar.rosen@skane.se

intensive care, monitoring of the electrocortical activity should have a continuous, simple recording setup and a small number of recording electrodes. Furthermore, EEG features that are immediately relevant for clinical decisions should be continuously available at the bedside and easily interpreted by the attending physician day and night. Such techniques have been applied for a long time in intensive care and anesthesia. It has also been used in neonatal monitoring, usually derived from a spectral analysis by fast Fourier transform (FFT) and presented as compressed spectral arrays (CSA) or spectral edge frequency (SE) [4].

Amplitude-integrated electroencephalogram

Amplitude-integrated EEG (aEEG) is a technique for simplified EEG monitoring that has found an increasing clinical application in neonatal intensive care. Details of the processing of the EEG signal are given in Fig. 1 and as follows for implementation: (1) analog signal conditioning, HPF 0.16 Hz, LPF 500 Hz (6 dB); (2) analog to digital conversion, antialiazing filter 76 Hz (6 dB), output sampling rate 256 Hz; (3) montage calculation. For example, (P3-REF) − (P4-REF) = P3-P4; (4) aEEG filter (see Fig. 1A); (5) semilogarithmic compression (see Fig. 1B); (6) envelope detection (see Fig. 1C); (7) data drawn on screen, calibrated for 6 mm/minute or 30 mm/minute.

In principle, the aEEG technique extracts the activity centered on the alpha band before amplification. More specifically, the method is based on a time-compressed (usually 6 cm/h) semilogarithmic (linear 0–10 μV, logarithmic 10–100 μV) display of the peak-to peak amplitude values of EEG passed through an asymmetrical bandpass filter that strongly enhances higher over lower frequencies, with suppression of activity below 2 Hz and above 15 Hz. This approach minimizes artifacts from sources such as sweating, movement, muscle activity, and interference. The EEG of the neonate, especially the preterm infant, is characterized by intermittent bursts of high amplitude, intermixed with lower amplitude continuous activity (Fig. 2). The bandwidth of the aEEG curve reflects variations in minimum and maximum EEG amplitude. The semilogarithmic display enhances identification of changes in the low voltage range and avoids overloading of the display at high amplitudes.

The cerebral function monitor (CFM) was designed in the 1960s by Maynard and originally applied in adult intensive care by Prior [5]. The method was first used in newborn babies in the late 1970s and early 1980s [6]. The CFM concept has been implemented in several new machines, based on digital technique and inverse digital reconstruction of the performance of the original CFM. In addition to the aEEG trend, these devices display the original EEG signal in present and past time, which is crucial for easier recognition of seizure patterns and artifacts. Published reports on neonatal aEEG include clinical and experimental studies [7,8]. The finding that the

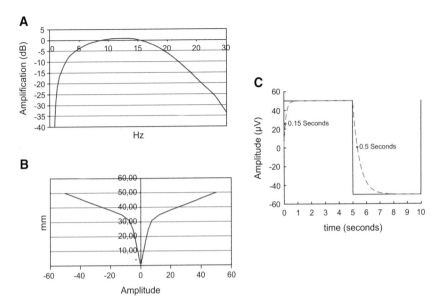

Fig. 1. (*A*) aEEG filter properties; (*B*) aEEG semilogarithmic scaling properties; (*C*) envelope onset and offset time properties. (*Data courtesy of* Viasys Healthcare, Inc., Conshohocken, Pennsylvania.)

information displayed by the aEEG paradigm can predict outcome after perinatal asphyxia is presently being used as an inclusion criterion in studies of therapeutic hypothermia [9]. The clinical experiences with neonatal aEEG monitoring have been summarized in an atlas [10].

For new users of aEEG, the value of the method is usually apparent when clinical aEEG reveals abnormal brain activity patterns that would otherwise pass unrecognized, such as subclinical seizure activity or deterioration caused by unexpected complications (eg, hypoglycemia or pneumothorax) [10]. It is, however, important to be aware of limitations and risks of over-interpretation when using aEEG [11,12]. The possibility of extracting de-tailed information is lost in exchange for markedly improved observation of long-term trends and changes in the overall cerebroelectrical activity. Therefore, continuous aEEG does not replace, but is complementary to, standard EEG. At least one standard EEG, preferably including a period of quiet sleep, should be recorded in infants monitored with aEEG.

Background electroencephalogram as reflected in amplitude integrated electroencephalogram

With the development of the cerebral connections during the first 20 to 45 weeks' postmenstrual age, the sources of spontaneous and synchronized neuronal activity, as reflected in the EEG, changes dramatically [13]. In

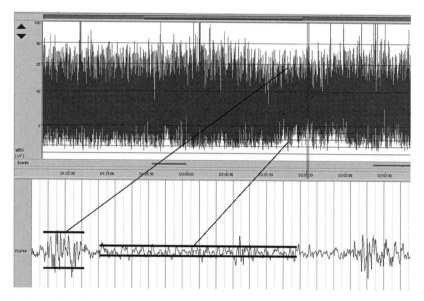

Fig. 2. aEEG and original EEG recording of discontinuous EEG. The peak-to-peak amplitude of the EEG bursts is defining the upper edge of the aEEG trace, and the peak to peak amplitude of the interburst EEG activity is defining the lower edge of the trace.

the preterm infant, the EEG pattern is dominated by slow activity transients (SAT) with superimposed higher-frequency oscillations [14]. The intervals between bursts gradually decrease with increasing gestational age (GA). The duration of continuous EEG activity between bursts gradually increases with GA and with the development of the thalamocortical and corticocortical connections.

The normal aEEG pattern changes with gestational age [5,15–19]. As predicted from EEG, the aEEG in the preterm infant is mainly discontinuous and becomes gradually more continuous with increasing GA [1]. The normal discontinuous EEG in preterm infants, tracé discontinue, with low amplitude EEG activity between bursts, should be distinguished from the abnormal pattern burst suppression with inactive (isoelectric) interburst intervals [20]. This difference is often possible to distinguish in the aEEG trace: the tracé discontinue pattern has a more variable lower margin around 0 to 6 μV (Fig. 2), whereas the burst suppression pattern has a straight low margin at 0 to 1 μV (Fig. 3) [2,7].

Cyclic alteration in behavioral states is a well-known phenomenon in term and preterm infants. Although the exact correlations with sleep stages later in life are not fully delineated, these cyclic changes of behavior are also reflected in cyclic changes in the EEG patterns [2,21]. Cyclic variations in the aEEG background, presumably reflecting cyclic alterations between periods of quiet sleep and periods of active sleep/wakefulness, can be seen in well infants from around 26 to 27 weeks' gestation [22,23]. A recently published

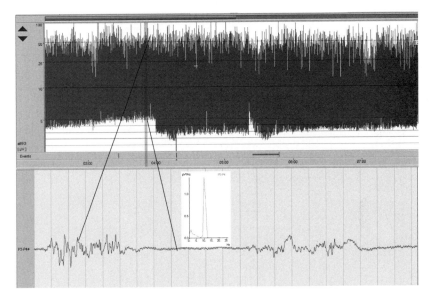

Fig. 3. aEEG and original EEG recording of a burst-suppression (BS) pattern. An artifact interference by high-frequency ventilator is indicated by a monorythmic activity at 11 Hz in the interburst intervals, which shifts the lower edge of the curve to a falsely high level.

study that evaluated sleep-wake cycling (SWC) in relation to standard EEG in stable preterm infants between 25 and 30 weeks supports the aEEG findings [24]. SWC develops with increasing maturation, and from 31 to 32 weeks' GA, quiet sleep periods are clearly discernable in the aEEG trace as distinct periods with increased bandwidth [16]. At term, these periods represent tracé alternant EEG patterns (Figs. 4 and 5).

The characterization of the background EEG activity may sometimes differ slightly between the aEEG and EEG. A discontinuous aEEG with low interburst amplitude at a level only slightly above zero may be classified as a burst-suppression pattern in the EEG [11]. This may be due to the high sensitivity of the aEEG in the low amplitude range. However, close inspection of the original EEG signal is necessary to exclude interference from electrocardiogram, electronic equipment, or high-frequency ventilation (Fig. 3).

Amplitude integrated electroencephalogram and acute metabolic failure

A critical breakdown of brain perfusion or energy metabolism immediately affects the amplitude of spontaneous or evoked EEG activity [7]. With a more gradual deterioration, such as hypoglycemia, the originally continuous EEG signal changes its frequency content and turns into a discontinuous suppression-bursts pattern before the EEG is abolished (Fig. 6) [25]. At restitution, the time course and degree of return of a normal

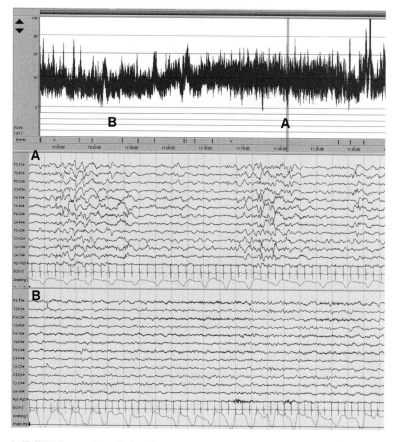

Fig. 4. Full EEG recording of a healthy term neonate during a full sleep cycle. A tracé alternant pattern is recorded in (B), and a continuous EEG during wakefulness in (A). The quiet sleep period is identified in the aEEG as a well-defined period of increased amplitude bandwidth.

EEG pattern reflects the extent of neuronal damage [26–28]. These experimental findings have been amply substantiated in many aEEG studies in infants after perinatal asphyxia and in adults after cardiac arrest and hypothermia [29–31].

Seizure patterns

In the aEEG, onset of seizure activity is usually seen as an abrupt increase of maximal and minimal aEEG amplitude, sometimes only minimal amplitude, often followed by a transient postictal amplitude depression (Fig. 7C). Single seizures are difficult to discriminate from a period of movement artifacts or a bad electrode from the aEEG trace, and a close inspection of the original EEG signal at the event is necessary (Fig. 7A). Occasionally

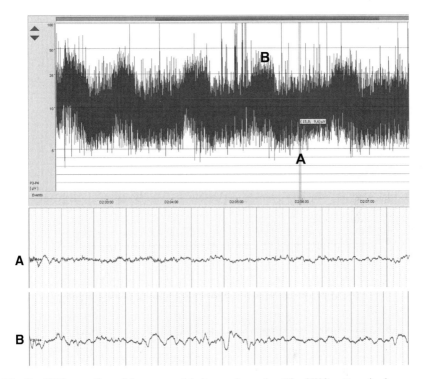

Fig. 5. aEEG recording of five sequential sleep-wake cycles. The SWC pattern is shown as repeated periods of increased amplitude variation as also shown in the original EEG records. A, quiet sleep; B, awake.

occurring seizures, especially those with short duration, are also easy to miss without an accompanying original EEG record (Fig. 8). Repeated seizures are identified as repeated peaks in the aEEG trace, sometimes described as a "sawtooth pattern" (Fig. 9). The appearance of a sawtooth pattern in the aEEG trace can also facilitate identification of an unclear rhythmic EEG pattern as an ictal EEG phenomenon (Fig. 10). The background EEG activity also affects the ease with which seizure patterns are discriminated in the aEEG trace. With a highly abnormal flat or discontinuous background, the onset of seizures is often more easily discernible than with a normal continuous EEG background [10]. Continuous spiking will not cause any abrupt changes of the aEEG trace, and would be missed in an aEEG record without access to the original EEG trace [32].

Concerns have been raised that with one single biparietal recording channel or with only one centroparietal channel on each side, focal seizures would be missed entirely by aEEG monitoring. In an early investigation, all seizures with duration more than 30 seconds, recorded simultaneously in five-channel tape-recorded EEG, could also be identified in a single-channel biparietal aEEG/CFM recording [32]. This may be explained by the fact

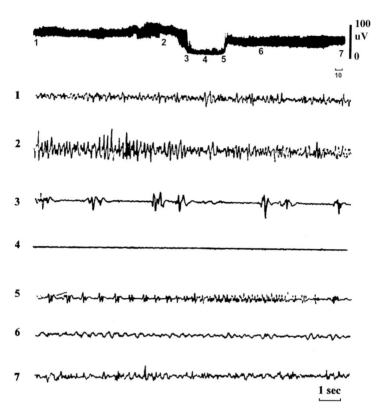

Fig. 6. Comparison of a continuous aEEG recording and samples of original EEG recorded from a rat before, during, and after a period of severe hypoglycemia induced by insulin given intraperitoneally. The blood glucose level was restored by intravenous glucose. (1) Normal EEG pattern. (2) Increased amplitude/decreased mean frequency. (3) Burst-suppression pattern. (4) Electrocortical inactivity. (5) Short electrographical seizure. (6) Continuous EEG of low amplitude. (7) Near-normal EEG pattern. (*Data from* Agardh CD, Rosén I. Neurophysiological recovery after hypoglycemic coma in the rat: correlation with cerebral metabolism. J Cereb Blood Flow Metab 1983;3:78–85.)

that although most neonatal seizures are focal in nature, the electrical fields evoked over the skull by the focal discharges are widely spread as a result of the volume conduction properties of the brain. This implies that these fields can be detected from electrode pairs distant from the electrical current sources, provided that the distance between the recording electrodes is kept large. This finding is illustrated in Fig. 11. In this case, three different focal seizures were recorded within a short time from the same infant, and the aEEG traces from the three commonly used aEEG leads were reconstructed. As can be seen, all three seizure discharges evoked widespread electrical fields, and all three seizures were detected in the biparietal lead. Similar to what has been described by Toet and colleagues [11], the case illustrates

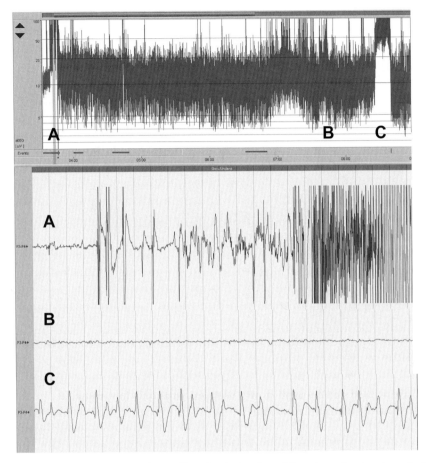

Fig. 7. aEEG and original EEG recording of a single seizure (C) as shown by abrupt onset of rhythmic seizure EEG pattern that causes a sudden upward shift of minimum and maximum aEEG amplitude. Checking the concomitant EEG makes it possible to safely discriminate this epileptic episode from an artifact caused by movement or a bad electrode (A). The low-amplitude interburst EEG is shown in (B).

that with a two-channel aEEG recording, focal seizures may appear more clearly in one unilateral channel than in the contralateral channel. Furthermore, in the author's experience, patients displaying focal seizures that are difficult to discriminate in the aEEG trace usually develop more widespread seizure patterns, which are easily detectable during the course of continuous monitoring.

Although some focal, low amplitude, and brief seizures may undoubtedly be missed, especially when only the aEEG trace without the concominant original EEG is available, it does not seem to create a major clinical problem in interpretation (see Refs. [11,12,32,33]).

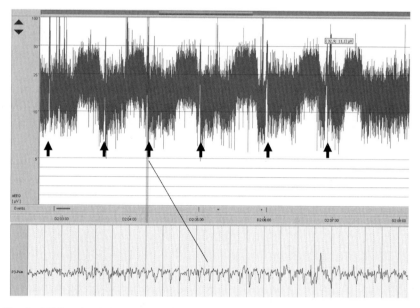

Fig. 8. aEEG and original EEG recording of a newborn with short electrographic seizures (*arrows*) when awakening from quiet sleep periods. In the aEEG trace the seizures are seen as abrupt increases of the minimum amplitude level. The epileptic nature of the episodes is confirmed in the original EEG.

Classification and description of a neonatal amplitude integrated electroencephalogram recording

aEEG tracings have been described and classified in several different ways, depending on whether normal or abnormal features have been addressed, and whether full-term or preterm infants have been in focus.

Amplitude integrated electroencephalogram in normal Infants

Many publications have described normal aEEG patterns in full-term and preterm infants (see Refs. [6,15–19]). Among the earlier studies, Verma and colleagues [15] and Viniker and colleagues [6] found that the aEEG feature most clearly related to maturation in healthy infants was the lower edge (amplitude) of the quiet sleep trace. In 1990, Thornberg and Thiringer [16] presented a study on normal aEEG development in preterm and full-term infants who had an uneventful neonatal period and were neurologically normal at follow-up; normative data for minimum and maximum amplitudes during wakefulness and sleep were presented. Burdjalov and colleagues [17] studied 30 infants with GA 24 to 39 weeks serially on 146 occasions, twice during the first 3 days of life and then weekly or biweekly. A scoring system was developed, evaluating continuity, cyclic (SWC) changes, amplitude of lower border, and bandwidth. The range of summarized score points

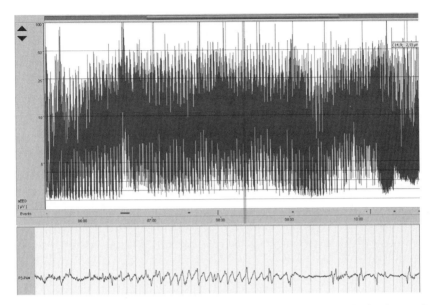

Fig. 9. aEEG and original EEG recording from a newborn with a status epilepticus/sawtooth pattern produced by recurrent short seizures of approximately 25 s duration. Each seizure causes an abrupt increase of minimum and maximum amplitude and a postictal depression of the minimum amplitude. The epileptic nature of the episodes is confirmed by inspection of the original EEG trace.

was 0 to 13. The total score correlated with gestational and postconceptional ages, and the highest total scores were attained at 35 to 36 weeks' postconceptional age gestation. Abnormal patterns (eg, burst suppression or seizures) were not included in the scoring system. Olischar and colleagues [18] recorded preterm infants, born at 23 to 29 gestational weeks and without cerebral ultrasound abnormalities, and defined quantitatively three different patterns: discontinuous low voltage, continuous, and discontinuous high voltage. Further normative data have recently been collected by Sisman and colleagues [19] from preterm infants without neurologic abnormalities who were born at 25 to 32 gestational weeks. Recordings were obtained biweekly from 24 to 48 hours of age until 35 postmenstrual weeks. Amplitude data largely substantiated those of Thornberg and Thiringer [16], and clear SWC was present from 29 gestational weeks.

Amplitude integrated electroencephalogram in infants with compromised brain function

Several studies have addressed and characterized abnormal aEEG records. Bjerre and colleagues [33] in one of the earlier studies described background patterns as continuous or interrupted (discontinuous). The recorded infants included asphyxiated preterm infants, full-term asphyxiated infants,

604   ROSÉN

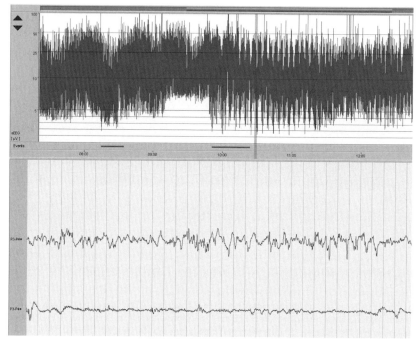

Fig. 10. aEEG and original EEG record of an episode, 1.5 h duration, with a sawtooth pattern indicating recurrent seizure activity. The aEEG pattern significantly contributes to the identification of seizures in this case where the original EEG is less obviously epileptic in character.

and infants up to 5 months who had suffered apparent life-threatening events. Cerebral recovery was associated with an initial continuous tracing or a change in background pattern from interrupted to continuous within 1 to 2 days of the hypoxic-ischemic insult. Hellström-Westas and colleagues [34] classified aEEG from asphyxiated full-term infants as continuous normal voltage (CNV), burst suppression (BS), continuous extremely low voltage (CLV), and flat (FT). Toet and colleagues [29] used a similar classification with the addition of discontinuous normal voltage (DNV) to the previous four patterns. Both classifications showed a high correlation with outcome. Infants with CNV or DNV during the first 6 hours of life were likely to survive without sequelae, whereas infants with BS, CLV, or FT had a high risk for death or severe handicap. Al Naqeeb and colleagues [35] used a classification including three categories for normal and abnormal aEEGs in full-term infants based on median upper and lower margin amplitude of the widest band of the aEEG trace. The aEEG background activity was classified as normal amplitude when the upper margin was greater than 10 μV and the lower margin was less than 5 μV; moderately abnormal when the upper margin was greater than 10 μV and the lower margin was less than 5μV; and suppressed when the upper margin was greater than 10 μV and the

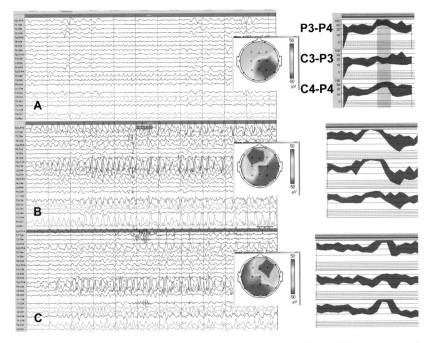

Fig. 11. Full EEG recordings of three focal seizures in an infant during aEEG monitoring. The seizures were predominantly frontal (A), one left-sided (B) and one right-sided (C). All three seizures produced widespread voltage gradients over the skull and caused clear-cut deflections in the P3-P4 aEEG derivation. Lateralized aEEG recordings showed according asymmetries. For further discussion, see text.

lower margin was less than 5 μV. Seizure activity was defined, but not sleep-wake cycling. This classification was recently used in a randomized multicenter study on postasphyxial head cooling. The intervention improved outcome in infants with a moderately abnormal aEEG pattern before 5.5 hours [9].

Recovery over time was a general feature of electrocortical background abnormalities after an insult. A few full-term postasphyxial infants with CLV/FT or BS patterns at 6 hours attained a CNV pattern within 24 hours, and half of them survived without sequelae [36].

Proposal for a new classification

Several models for classification of aEEG patterns have been suggested. It is obvious that some classifications are relevant only for a certain group of NICU patients (eg, asphyxiated full-term or normal preterm infants). Therefore, a new classification of aEEG background patterns is proposed based on EEG terminology, which could be used in all newborn infants (Box 1) [37]. In this proposal, some of the classifications described previously have been used or modified. The classification does not include evaluation of

Box 1. Suggested classification of amplitude integrated electroencephalogram patterns in preterm and term infants

Background pattern describes the dominating type of electro-cortical activity in the aEEG trace.

- Continuous (C): continuous activity with lower (minimum) amplitude around (5)–7–10 μV and maximum amplitude 10–25(–50) μV.
- Discontinuous (DC): discontinuous background with minimum amplitude variable, but below 5 μV, and maximum amplitude above 10 μV.
- Continuous low voltage (CLV): continuous background pattern of low voltage (around or below 5 μV).
- Burst suppression (BS): discontinuous background with minimum amplitude without variability at 0–1(2) μV, and bursts with amplitude greater than 25 μV. BS+ denotes burst density 100 or more bursts/h, and BS– means burst density less than 100 bursts/h.
- Inactive, flat (FT): mainly inactive (isoelectric tracing) background below 5 μV.

Sleep-wake cycling
Sleep-wake cycling (SWC) in the aEEG is characterized by smooth sinusoidal variations, mainly in the minimum amplitude. The broader bandwidth represents discontinuous background activity during quiet sleep (tracé alternant EEG in term infants), and the more narrow bandwidth corresponds to more continu-ous activity during wakefulness and active sleep.

- No SWC: no cyclic variation of the aEEG background.
- Imminent/immature SWC: some, but not fully developed, cyclic variation of the lower amplitude, but not developed as compared with normative gestational age representative data.
- Developed SWC: clearly identifiable sinusoidal variations between discontinuous and more continuous background activity with cycle duration 20 or more minutes.

Seizures
Epileptic seizure activity in the aEEG is usually seen as an abrupt rise in the minimum amplitude, usually accompanied by a rise in the maximum amplitude. The raw EEG should show simulta-neous seizure activity with a gradual build-up and then decline, in frequency and amplitude, of repetitive spikes or sharp wave or activity with duration at least 5 to 10 s.

- Single: a solitary seizure.
- Repetitive: single seizures appearing more frequently than at 30-min intervals.
- Status epilepticus: continuously ongoing seizure activity greater than 30 min.

background patterns and amplitudes in relation to normative data for different gestational ages. Many EEG terms (eg, focal, multifocal, sharp waves, delta pattern) are not relevant for aEEG, as a trend monitor does not provide this type of information. Similar to basic EEG interpretation, pattern recognition forms the basis also for interpretation of the aEEG trace (Fig. 12).

The amplitude of the electrocortical activity is important, but this measure must be handled with caution, as voltage may be affected by interelectrode distance and scalp edema. Furthermore, extracerebral signals like electrocardiogram and high-frequency oscillation ventilation may significantly interfere with the interpretation of a discontinuous signal as DNV versus BS or LV versus FT (Fig. 3). Close inspection of the original EEG trace accompanying the aEEG trace in modern equipment is highly recommended. Nevertheless, normative values for minimum and maximum amplitudes of the aEEG at different gestational ages have been published and are helpful

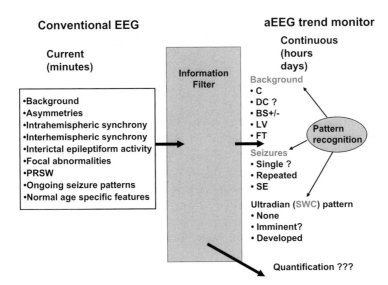

Fig. 12. Conceptual view of the aEEG as compared with EEG. aEEG helps in continuously extracting three features—background activity, sleep-wake cycling, and seizure pattern—that have been proven to be relevant for prognosis and treatment of the preterm newborn and ill newborn.

for assisting in evaluating aEEG recordings in relation to normal traces for a certain gestational age (see Refs. [6,15,16,19]). The minimum amplitude at quiet sleep periods is especially valuable to assess, as it increases with gestational age up to term. Furthermore, short-time variability of minimum amplitude is a sign that separates a discontinuous EEG from a BS pattern.

Summary

aEEG is a method for continuous long-term monitoring of brain activity that has proved to be successful in newborn infants of all gestational ages, and that will probably gain more widespread use in NICUs. The simplicity of the method makes it possible to apply and interpret around the clock by the neonatal staff, and the interinterpreter reliability is usually excellent (see Refs. [11,30,35,38]). Because of the small number of electrodes, single-channel biparietal aEEG is also practical for monitoring the most preterm infants.

A common classification of patterns would be beneficial and increase understanding of the method. Many studies have shown that the previously used classifications are relevant for identifying abnormalities that could lead to early intervention. They have been designed for special purposes and are not generally applicable to all clinical situations. The three main features that can be extracted from neonatal aEEGs—background activity, SWC, and electrographic seizure patterns—reflect different physiologic and pathophysiologic mechanisms with different clinical implications in various groups of infants and should be described separately (Fig. 12). We are therefore not suggesting an overall rating score for clinical aEEG.

The aEEG also identifies subclinical seizure activity that would otherwise pass without detection. In this context, however, users of aEEG must be aware that although seizure identification with a single- or two-channel monitor is valuable, some seizures may pass unrecognized. Brief, single, and focal seizures, in particular, as well as continuous spiking, may be missed by inspection of the aEEG trace only. In the author's experience, the additional display of the original EEG signal provided in modern devices improves the sensitivity and makes it possible to discriminate single seizures from periods of artifacts due to patient care procedures, for example. Close collaboration with neurologists and neurophysiologists is recommended and such collaboration is made easier when the recording equipment can be connected to a hospital network. Standard EEGs should be recorded frequently in infants undergoing aEEG, especially when an abnormal pattern is noted.

An important issue is how many channels of EEG should be integrated into aEEG traces. For standard monitoring, one or two channels are probably sufficient. When abnormalities are identified and localized in standard EEG, the number and positioning of aEEG recordings may be modified. With a bilateral two-channel aEEG monitor, one may be able to identify

gross asymmetries in background and seizure patterns (Fig. 11) [11]. These types of findings should be substantiated by multichannel standard EEG to make certain that the asymmetry is not the result of an artifact. A multichannel system as standard monitoring is not usually feasible because it may hinder the care and disturb the patient, which is especially relevant for the fragile preterm infant.

The CFM paradigm for aEEG was developed by Maynard and Prior for use in adult intensive care but has been found to be useful also in neonatal EEG monitoring. This technology would probably have been different, however, if it had been developed de novo for neonatal applications. Probably the ideal EEG trend monitor for neonatal use has yet to be developed. The addition of an original EEG trace is of significant value. Calculation of burst density from aEEG traces of discontinuous EEG is tedious and should be replaced by a direct additional trend displaying bursts per hour or interburst interval. Furthermore, spectral content of the EEG expressed as, for example, spectral edge frequency has been found to be of relevance in experimental and clinical studies of white matter injury in premature infants [4,39]. The spectral content of bursts of discontinuous EEG under normal and abnormal conditions may turn out to provide clinical useful information [40]. Recent studies show that low-frequency (DC) components are predominant in the immature EEG and may become relevant to include in future continuous monitoring paradigms [14,41]. Automatic seizure detection is an issue that is currently explored. EEG trend analysis may be combined in integrated systems with other modalities, such as near infrared spectroscopy, for continuous evaluation of brain function in sick neonates.

In conclusion, aEEG has become a standard method for simple brain monitoring in neonatal intensive care. The aEEG is derived from the original EEG signal in a well-defined way, by reverse engineering copying the performance of the CFM machine originally developed by Maynard and Prior. Several instruments are available that provide the aEEG signal with slightly different displays. After some training, a user can classify hours of aEEG recording according to background activity, presence of seizures, and sleep-wake cycling to make clinical decisions based on a large body of evidence from studies in newborn babies. This makes around-the-clock brain monitoring possible in every neonatal intensive care unit. New digital instruments provide access to the original EEG signal and alternate ways of trend analysis. Further research will show if these options are clinically useful.

References

[1] Connell JA, Oozeer R, Dubowitz V. Continuous 4-channel EEG monitoring: a guide to interpretation, with normal values, in preterm infants. Neuropediatrics 1987;18:138–45.
[2] Lamblin MD, Andre M, Challamel MJ, et al. Electroencephalography of the premature and term newborn. Maturational aspects and glossary. Neurophysiol Clin 1999;29: 123–219.

[3] Holmes GL, Lombroso CT. Prognostic value of background patterns in the neonatal EEG. J Clin Neurophysiol 1993;10:323–52.

[4] Inder TE, Buckland L, Williams CE, et al. Lowered electroencephalographic spectral edge frequency predicts the presence of cerebral white matter injury in premature infants. Pediatrics 2003;111:27–33.

[5] Maynard D, Prior PF, Scott DF. Device for continuous monitoring of cerebral activity in resuscitated patients. BMJ 1969;4:545–6.

[6] Viniker DA, Maynard DE, Scott DF. Cerebral function monitor studies in neonates. Clin Electroencephalogr 1984;15:185–92.

[7] Bunt JE, Gavilanes AW, Reulen JP, et al. The influence of acute hypoxemia and hypovolemic hypotension on neuronal brain activity measured by the cerebral function monitor in new-born piglets. Neuropediatrics 1996;27:260–4.

[8] de Vries LS, Hellstrom-Westas L. Role of cerebral function monitoring in the newborn. Arch Dis Child Fetal Neonatal Ed 2005;90:F201–7.

[9] Gluckman PD, Wyatt JS, Azzopardi D, et al. Selective head cooling with mild systemic hypothermia after neonatal encephalopathy: multicentre randomised trial. Lancet 2005;365: 663–70.

[10] Hellström-Westas L, de Vries LS, Rosén I. An atlas of amplitude-integrated EEGs in the newborn. London: Parthenon Publishing; 2003.

[11] Toet MC, van der Meij W, de Vries LS, et al. Comparison between simultaneously recorded amplitude integrated EEG (cerebral function monitor) and standard EEG in neonates. Pediatrics 2002;109:772–9.

[12] Rennie JM, Chorley G, Boylan GB, et al. Non-expert use of the cerebral function monitor for neonatal seizure detection. Arch Dis Child Fetal Neonatal Ed 2004;89:F37–40.

[13] Kostovic I, Jovanov-Milosevic N. The development of cerebral connections during the first 20–45 weeks' gestation. Semin Neonatol, in press.

[14] Vanhatalo S, Tallgren P, Andersson S, et al. DC-EEG discloses prominent, very slow wave activity patterns during sleep in preterm infants. Clin Neurophysiol 2002;113:1822–5.

[15] Verma UL, Archbald F, Tejani N, et al. Cerebral function monitor in the neonate. I. Normal patterns. Dev Med Child Neurol 1984;26:154–61.

[16] Thornberg E, Thiringer K. Normal patterns of cerebral function monitor traces in term and preterm neonates. Acta Paediatr Scand 1990;79:20–5.

[17] Burdjalov VF, Baumgart S, Spitzer AR. Cerebral function monitoring: a new scoring system for the evaluation of brain maturation in neonates. Pediatrics 2003;112:855–61.

[18] Olischar M, Klebermass K, Kuhle S, et al. Reference values for amplitude-integrated electroencephalographic activity in preterm infants younger than 30 weeks' gestational age. Pediatrics 2004;113:e61–6.

[19] Sisman J, Campbell DE, Brion LP. Amplitude-integrated EEG in preterm infants: maturation of background pattern and amplitude voltage with postmenstrual age and gestational age. J Perinatol 2005;25:391–6.

[20] Lombroso CT. Neonatal polygraphy in full-term and premature infants: a review of normal and abnormal findings. J Clin Neurophysiol 1985;2:105–55.

[21] Blumberg MS, Lucas DE. A developmental and component analysis of active sleep. Dev Psychobiol 1996;29(1):1–22.

[22] Hellström-Westas L, Rosen I, Svenningsen NW. Cerebral function monitoring during the first week of life in extremely small low birthweight (ESLBW) infants. Neuropediatrics 1991;22:27–32.

[23] Kuhle S, Klebermass K, Olischar M, et al. Sleep-wake cycles in preterm infants below 30 weeks of gestational age. Preliminary results of a prospective amplitude-integrated EEG study. Wien Klin Wochenschr 2001;113:219–23.

[24] Scher MS, Johnson MW, Holditch-Davis D. Cyclicity of neonatal sleep behaviors at 25 to 30 weeks' postconceptional age. Pediatr Res 2005;57:879–82.

[25] Agardh CD, Rosén I. Neurophysiological recovery after hypoglycemic coma in the rat: correlation with cerebral metabolism. J Cereb Blood Flow Metab 1983;3:78–85.

[26] Hossmann KA, Kleihues P. Reversibility of ischemic brain damage. Arch Neurol 1973;29: 375–82.

[27] Rehncrona S, Rosén I, Smith ML. Effect of different degrees of brain ischemia and tissue lactic acidosis on the short-term recovery of neurophysiological and metabolic variables. Exp Neurol 1985;87:458–73.

[28] Rosén I, Smith ML, Rehncrona S. Quantitative EEG and evoked potentials after experimental brain ischemia in the rat; correlation with cerebral metabolism and blood flow. Prog Brain Res 1984;63:175–83.

[29] Toet MC, Hellström-Westas L, Groenendaal F, et al. Amplitude integrated EEG 3 and 6 hours after birth in full term neonates with hypoxic-ischaemic encephalopathy. Arch Dis Child Fetal Neonatal Ed 1999;81:F19–23.

[30] Thorngren-Jerneck K, Hellstrom-Westas L, Ryding E, et al. Cerebral glucose metabolism and early EEG/aEEG in term newborn infants with hypoxic-ischemic encephalopathy. Pediatr Res 2003;54:854–60.

[31] Rundgren M, Rosén I, Friberg H. Amplitude-integrated EEG (aEEG) predicts outcome after cardiac arrest and induced hypothermia. Intensive Care Med, in press.

[32] Hellstrom-Westas L. Comparison between tape-recorded and amplitude-integrated EEG monitoring in sick newborn infants. Acta Paediatr Scand 1992;81:812–9.

[33] Bjerre I, Hellström-Westas L, Rosén I, et al. Monitoring of cerebral function after severe birth asphyxia in infancy. Arch Dis Child 1983;58:997–1002.

[34] Hellström-Westas L, Rosén I, Svenningsen NW. Predictive value of early continuous amplitude integrated EEG recordings on outcome after severe birth asphyxia in full term infants. Arch Dis Child 1995;72:F34–8.

[35] Al Naqeeb N, Edwards AD, Cowan F, et al. Assessment of neonatal encephalopathy by amplitude integrated electroencephalography. Pediatrics 1999;103:1263–71.

[36] van Rooij LG, Toet MC, Osredkar D, et al. Recovery of amplitude integrated electroencephalographic background patterns within 24 hours of perinatal asphyxia. Arch Dis Child Fetal Neonatal Ed 2005;90:F245–51.

[37] Hellström-Westas L, Rosén I, de Vries LS, et al. Amplitude integrated EEG: classification and interpretation in preterm and term infants. Neoreviews 2006;7:e76–87.

[38] ter Horst HJ, Sommer C, Bergman KA, et al. Prognostic significance of amplitude-integrated EEG during the first 72 hours after birth in severely asphyxiated neonates. Pediatr Res 2004;55:1026–33.

[39] Fraser M, Bennet L, Gunning M, et al. Cortical electroencephalogram suppression is associated with post-ischemic cortical injury in 0.65 gestation fetal sheep. Brain Res Dev Brain Res 2005;154:45–55.

[40] Thordstein M, Flisberg A, Löfgren N, et al. Spectral analysis of burst periods in EEG from healthy and post-asphyctic full-term neonates. Clin Neurophysiol 2004;115:2462–6.

[41] Vanhatalo S, Palva M, Andersson S, et al. Slow endogenous activity transients and developmental expression of K+-Cl-cotransporter 2 in the immature human cortex. Eur J Neurosci 2005;22:2799–804.

ELSEVIER
SAUNDERS

CLINICS IN
PERINATOLOGY

Clin Perinatol 33 (2006) 613–618

Brain Monitoring in the Neonate—the Rationale

Gorm Greisen, MD, DMSc

Department of Neonatology, 5024 Rigshospitalet, Blegdamsvej 9, 2100 Copenhagen, Denmark

Imagine a 25-week-old baby, just delivered because of cervical insufficiency. Her brain weighs just more than 100 g and is presumably normal, but is nonetheless very immature. How can it be protected and supported to grow and develop normally? What role does modern cerebral monitoring play in this process? Currently, the answer is probably none. This article analyzes the reasons and points out some areas of potential that may have future benefits.

Monitoring to allow timely intervention

Monitoring means using oversight to detect threats early enough for effective intervention. It permits timely intervention to avoid potentially harmful consequences. Apnea detection is a prime example. Because it is a frequent problem in preterm babies, some type of monitoring would very likely be part of our hypothetical patient's standard care. Apnea can cause death or damage, and intervention is usually very effective in preventing associated problems. Since the timescale of apnea is on the order of seconds to minutes, an apnea alarm must always be audible, and the person hearing it must know what to do and be able to it without delay. Because of the pathophysiology of apnea, and for technological reasons, modern medical practice often detects apnea through ECG monitoring or pulse oximetry. Decreases in either the oxygen saturation or heart rate in an apneic infant result in immediate intervention when an event occurs. The value of monitoring in this situation is clear.

Monitoring of ischemia

One particular threat to our patient's brain, cerebral hypoxia caused by low blood flow, is similar to that seen in infants who have many different

---
E-mail address: greisen@rh.dk

primary problems, such as congenital heart disease, arterial hypotension, or low Pco_2. A blood flow below the level necessary to support normal function is called *ischemia*. Whether current monitoring methods can detect cerebral ischemia in a timely fashion to avoid further deterioration in cerebral function is a critical issue, because ischemia may interfere with brain growth and, when more severe, can cause brain damage.

Three candidate methods for monitoring cerebral ischemia are currently used: Doppler ultrasound, near-infrared spectroscopy (NIRS), and amplitude-integrated electroencephalogram (aEEG). These methods can be used to monitor flow, tissue oxygenation, and neuronal function. Why do these devices not sit on the head of every baby who is at-risk?

Monitoring of cerebral ischemia is not yet standard care in preterm babies for several reasons. Doppler ultrasound in intracranial arteries measures blood-flow velocity not blood flow, and Doppler ultrasound in the superior vena cava measures flow not only to the brain but also to the head, neck, and upper extremities. NIRS measures mixed vascular hemoglobin oxygen saturation, not tissue oxygenation. Normal ranges are wide and the relationships between flow, oxygenation, and function are weak. In addition, interventions to increase blood flow and tissue oxygenation are not well established and their value in effecting normalization of the EEG has not been studied systematically. Last, and perhaps most importantly, the clinical value of a package consisting of monitoring, an interpretation algorithm, and intervention has not yet been proven. Actually, there are doubts as to the importance of cerebral ischemia as a risk factor for brain damage and as a risk factor for neurodevelopmental deficit. Both are common in extremely preterm babies.

A lesson from obstetrics

A lesson on monitoring can be learned from the history of fetal ST-analysis (STAN [Neoventa, Mølndal, Sweden]), which is based on the fact that the myocardium is particularly exposed during episodes of fetal distress and that the increased extracellular $K+$ concentration induced by glycolysis in the myocardium is detectable as an ST-segment elevation [1]. Experts believed that monitoring in this situation would add to the (limited) capabilities of discrete auscultation and fetal heart rate monitoring in detecting progressive asphyxia during labor. STAN analysis could therefore be clinically important in detecting a fetus that had potential injury, and allow timely intervention and earlier delivery and reduce the number of inappropriate interventions that might occur because of the low specificity of an abnormal fetal heart rate tracing. Because severe birth asphyxia is a rare event, a large randomized controlled trial added STAN to fetal heart rate monitoring [2]. This trial showed the second benefit of STAN, which was reduced operative deliveries for fetal distress, but not the first, which was improved neurologic outcome. The technology, however, had been protected by patents. As a result, the next large industry-sponsored trial tested a package consisting of equipment, computer-assisted diagnostics, intervention algorithm, and personnel training, showing a clinical benefit in reduced risk for significant metabolic acidosis at birth [3] and reduced incidence of neonatal encephalopathy [4].

The STAN studies suggest that consistent interpretation of monitoring data and consistent use of appropriate interventions are prerequisites for a clinical benefit. Proving the benefit of a new diagnostic technique is as demanding as proving the benefit of a new drug.

The form of monitoring data

For monitoring of brain hypoxia, one aspect is straightforward. Cerebral venous oxygen saturation is a well-defined reference variable, with a value ranging between 0% and 100%. Normal values are typically 65% to 70% and the critical range is usually below 40% saturation. Experience from animal research and adult neuro-intensive care can be used to define an interval of normality and a threshold for intervention.

Other monitors do not have a well-defined reference variable. Although a descriptive study can define the interval of normality, or rather an interval of common values, it cannot define a threshold for intervention. For instance, subtle seizures are not normal, but whether intervention is beneficial in avoiding the long-term adverse effects is unclear.

Even when a threshold for intervention can be defined, the situation is more complex when data are continuous. Relevant questions are how far below the threshold and for how long does the abnormality exist. For ischemia (in adult brain), a few minutes of no flow can cause damage, whereas at 25% of normal blood flow injury may take an hour to occur. In STAN, the instrument identifies a time multiplied by severity integral and flags an event. This event is a precise trigger for the diagnostic process that helps decide whether the baby should be delivered emergently.

Added value

An important issue in monitoring is added value. This factor is often neglected when diagnostic methods are evaluated. Added value is what results from a new method when added to what is already known about the patient. Cerebral monitoring is not applied in isolation. Standard care of any infant also includes monitoring of oxygen saturation, blood gases, blood sugar, blood pressure, and numerous other clinical variables, such as color, spontaneous movements, and reactions to care. The function of other organs is indicated by monitoring of feeding tolerance, diuresis, blood coagulation, or liver enzymes. The question, therefore, is what value a brain monitoring method can add to this clinical context.

The operation of monitors

The technical complexity of monitoring modalities that clinical researchers can handle differs from what clinical staff can handle. Because clinical staff have less training, time, motivation, and knowledge, especially when new monitoring techniques are used, more errors will generally occur and more limited efforts will be made to sort out findings that are unclear. In clinical care, demanding diagnostic methods are left to specialized staff such as radiographers or electrophysiology technicians. For a method to be used consistently by nurses or physicians, the time and effort needed to understand the new device must be outweighed by the immediate, well-defined clinical benefit.

Monitoring to diagnose brain damage

Sequential brain ultrasound would be part of standard care for our hypothetical infant in most neonatal units. The purpose of ultrasound is to define the individual chance of normal neurodevelopmental outcome rather than diagnose a condition to be treated early. Intraventricular hemorrhage and periventricular leukomalacia, although ominous, are rarely treatable. They are diagnosed by ultrasound to better understand the potential long-term outcome in an infant. In many neonatal units, under certain conditions, the results may potentially contribute to a decision to withhold or withdraw life support. Here, timely intervention has a different meaning. Therefore, cerebral monitoring in certain situations may be valuable, whereas in others, additional information must still be elicited and further research required.

Other monitoring methods, such as aEEG or sequential MRI, may help predict an unacceptable outcome. Only rarely have they shown added value in systematic studies. An exception is when an aEEG is performed 3 to 6 hours after birth in a term baby with neonatal encephalopathy.

Brain monitoring for research

Brain monitoring research is typically nontherapeutic, with a primary purpose of studying disease processes. For example, the study of germinal layer hemorrhage and the focus on the vulnerability of the cerebral circulation in newborns have led to more careful management of very preterm babies. Although the history is not straightforward regarding progress in this area, the discovery of the high prevalence of cerebral hemorrhage in the late 1970s and the studies on cerebral blood flow during the 1980s were followed by a decrease in the overall prevalence of cerebral hemorrhage. Similarly, the link between periventricular leukomalacia and cerebral palsy and hyperventilation/hypocapnia seems to have decreased this risk factor.

One particular ethical problem may be that nontherapeutic research is often crucially important and may be even more important compared with therapeutic research. Once disease processes are better understood, monitoring and prevention may be possible. In the usual ethical arguments, nontherapeutic research should only be performed in children if the risks are negligible (ie, comparable to those of common daily life). The fundamental belief is that when a research project has no potential benefit to the participant (as opposed to the circumstances in therapeutic trials), it takes a motive of altruism to consent, and although competent individuals can decide this for themselves, parents cannot decide that their children should be altruistic.

Strictly speaking, however, nontherapeutic research may have some potential benefit for participants. Many monitoring methods do provide information that may be useful, if made immediately available to the caring clinician. For instance, the clinician and parents may feel reassured if experimental monitoring shows nothing abnormal. Such reassurance may be even more valuable if the infant is ill.

Is this a paradox, however? How can one feel reassured by a normal result if no brain monitoring in the neonate has been documented to improve outcome? Or, is the number of times one can feel reassured by normal results outweighed by the number of times one can feel upset by abnormal results? If normal results are more common than abnormal ones, then good news is actually not much news at all.

In the author's opinion, people value knowledge even when it is of no immediate use to them. Most people prefer to know rather than stay uninformed about important issues. Assuming that researchers are appropriately modest about the accuracy and significance of the findings, the little knowledge provided may allow the caring clinician and parents to form a somewhat clearer picture of the baby's actual clinical situation. This phenomenon could be called the *optimism bias* in knowledge, whereby people insist that they may, in some way, gain from it. This line of thought may be an ethical defense for continued research into brain monitoring in neonates.

An optimistic note

The high prevalence of neurodevelopmental deficits in children born preterm provides a clear rationale about the relevance and importance of cerebral monitoring. Because of the complexity of the brain, and the even greater complexity of brain development in a process of interaction with a complex environment, studying causation is extraordinarily difficult.

Knowledge of a causation is necessary for specific prevention. One method is to break up the process and study some of its parts, and current brain monitoring, especially the new and more ingenious approaches, will likely be most helpful. Establishing causation between modifiable factors and brain dysfunction or damage is most important. For this purpose, methods need not be suitable for clinical routine or be cost-effective; they only need to be reliable and used in a sound research context.

Summary

Experts argue that no brain monitoring of clinical value is currently available for the very preterm baby. Evidence is lacking about all parts of the therapeutic package: specificity and sensitivity for severe brain compromise, effectiveness of specific intervention, and overall clinical value over and above standard care. However, brain monitoring will probably be most important ultimately for establishing specific causation between modifiable factors and brain dysfunction or damage.

References

[1] Hokegard KH, Karlsson K, Kjellmer I, et al. ECG-changes in the fetal lamb during asphyxia in relation to beta-adrenoceptor stimulation and blockade. Acta Physiol Scand 1979;105: 195–203.
[2] Westgate J, Harris M, Curnow JSH, et al. Plymouth randomized trial of cardiotocogram only versus ST waveform plus cardiotocogram for intrapartum monitoring: 2,400 cases. Am J Obstet Gynecol 1993;169:1151–60.
[3] Amer-Wåhlin I, Hellsten C, Norén H, et al. Cardiotocography only versus cardiotocography plus ST analysis of fetal electrocardiogram for intrapartum fetal monitoring: a Swedish randomised controlled trial. Lancet 2001;358:534–8.
[4] Norén H, Amer-Wåhlin I, Hagberg H, et al. Fetal electrocardiography in labor and neonatal outcome: data from the Swedish randomized controlled trial on intrapartum fetal monitoring. Am J Obstet Gynecol 2003;188:183–92.

CLINICS IN
PERINATOLOGY

Clin Perinatol 33 (2006) 619–632

Amplitude Integrated Electroencephalography in the Full-Term Newborn

Linda S. de Vries, MD, PhD*, Mona C. Toet, MD, PhD

Department of Neonatology, KE 04.123.1, Wilhelmina Children's Hospital,
University Medical Center, P.O. Box 85090, 3508 AB Utrecht, the Netherlands

Approximately 10 to 15 years ago, few centers in the world used continuous electroencephalography (EEG) monitoring in full-term newborns admitted with neonatal encephalopathy (NE) or seizures. The absence of neurologic monitoring contrasted greatly with monitoring of respiratory rate, heart rate, ECG, oxygen saturation, and blood pressure, which were all well integrated into the routine care of any newborn infant admitted to a neonatal intensive care unit (NICU). When clinical seizures were suspected, a standard EEG would be performed and, if seizures were detected, treatment initiated with phenobarbitone and phenytoin, the most common antiepileptic drugs. The neurophysiologist would then assess the background pattern and the results would be considered in giving the prognosis. A few studies using video-EEG recordings have shown that the commonly used antiepileptic drugs are only effective in approximately half of the infants [1]. Furthermore, experts have increasingly recognized that subclinical seizures are very common, especially after antiepileptic drugs are administered [2,3].

The cerebral function monitor (CFM) was originally designed by Maynard in the late 1960s to perform continuous electrocortical monitoring [4]. The device was initially used to monitor adults during anesthesia and in intensive care after cardiac arrest, during status epilepticus, and after heart surgery [5,6]. In the early 1980s, the technique was introduced into neonatal intensive care [7–9] and experts quickly realized that long-term recordings in high-risk, full-term infants who had NE were especially interesting [7,9].

Dr. de Vries and Dr. Toet have been involved in the development or testing of the instruments (BrainZ, BrainZ instruments, Auckland, New Zealand; Olympic 6000; Olympic Medical, Seattle) from which records are shown in this article. They do not have an economic interest in the production or sales of these instruments.

* Corresponding author.
E-mail address: l.s.devries@umcutrecht.nl (L.S. de Vries).

doi:10.1016/j.clp.2006.06.002   *perinatology.theclinics.com*

The term *amplitude-integrated EEG* (aEEG) is currently preferred. The initial analog CFM device usually recorded a single channel from one pair of biparietally placed electrodes (corresponding to P_3 and P_4 according to the international EEG 10–20 classification, ground F_z). Since the introduction of the initial analog CFM device, several digital machines have become available, some able to record more than just a single channel. Using two channels provides information about hemispheric asymmetry, which may be helpful in children who have a unilateral brain lesion. The signal is amplified and passed through an asymmetric band-pass filter that strongly attenuates activity less than 2 Hz and more than 15 Hz to minimize artifacts from sources such as sweating, muscle activity, and electric interference. Additional processing includes semilogarithmic amplitude compression, rectification, and time compression. The signal is shown on paper or on the computer screen as a semilogarithmic scale at slow speed (6 cm/h) (Fig. 1). The electrode impedance is either shown continuously as a second tracing or as an alarm when the impedance is too high. The bandwidth in the output reflects variations in minimum and maximum EEG amplitude, which depend on the maturity and severity of illness of the newborn infant. Because of the semilogarithmic scale used to plot the output, changes in background activity of very low amplitude ($<5\mu V$) are enhanced.

Use of amplitude-integrated electroencephalography in neonatal encephalopathy

In full-term infants who have NE, who are often admitted at night or during the weekend, immediate access to aEEG monitoring is one of many advantages of this technique. aEEG is easy to learn for senior and junior doctors and the nursing staff and provides immediate information

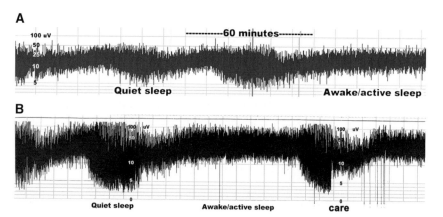

Fig. 1. (*A*) Normal continuous normal voltage background pattern with sleep–wake cycling in a full-term infant. (*B*) Acute disruption of quiet sleep by care in an infant of gestational age 35 weeks.

about the background activity and presence of seizures within hours after birth. This information is required as soon as possible after birth to select patients for neuroprotective intervention and predict neurodevelopmental outcome [10].

Assessment of amplitude-integrated electroencephalography background pattern

The value of the background pattern in the prediction of neurodevelopmental outcome was already well established with the use of the standard EEG [11]. A poor background pattern that persists beyond the first 12 to 24 hours after birth (burst suppression, low voltage, or flat trace) is well known to carry a poor prognosis. The interburst interval can be calculated and, using standard EEG, a study recently showed that a predominant duration of more than 30 seconds correlated with the occurrence of unfavorable neurologic outcome and subsequent epilepsy ($P = .040$ and $P = .033$, respectively) [12]. This predictive value has also been shown for the aEEG in several studies within 3 to 6 hours after birth [13–15]. A classification system based on pattern recognition [14,15] can be used or actual values of lower and upper margins of activity can be considered [16]. Although values rather than patterns may be preferred, values may be misleading because the voltage may be affected by interelectrode distance and scalp edema. The lower margin may also be elevated because of extracranial activity (eg, ECG interference or interference with a high-frequency ventilator [HFV]). This so-called "drift of the baseline" is particularly seen in infants who have a severely depressed background pattern (Fig. 2). The simultaneous recording of the real EEG, present on the newer digital devices, may help identify an ECG or HFV artifact. We therefore prefer using pattern recognition, also taking the values of upper and lower margins into account [17]. Hellström-Westas and colleagues [14] classified aEEG from asphyxiated full-term infants as continuous normal voltage (CNV), burst suppression, continuous extremely low voltage (CLV), and flat trace. Toet and colleagues [15] created a similar classification with five categories, adding discontinuous normal voltage (DNV) to the existing four patterns (Fig. 3). More recently, the different patterns of dominating electrocortical activity were slightly adjusted into five patterns, also taking the voltage into account [17]:

1. CNV: continuous activity with lower (minimum) amplitude around (5) to 7 to 10 μV and maximum amplitude 10 to 25 (−50) μV.
2. DNC: discontinuous background with minimum amplitude variable, but less than 5 μV, and maximum amplitude more than 10 μV.
3. Burst suppression: discontinuous background with minimum amplitude without variability at 0 to 1 (2) μV, and bursts with amplitude more than 25 μV.
4. CLV: continuous background pattern of very low voltage (around or below 5 μV).

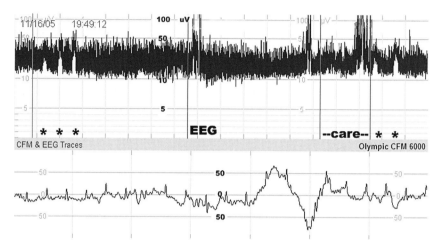

Fig. 2. Lower and upper margin of the band of aEEG activity are more than 10 μV. The "real EEG," however, shows a lot of ECG artifact, which could be held responsible for this "drift of the baseline" in the infant who has severe NE with an arterial lactate more than 30 mmol/L after resuscitation at birth. Also note repetitive ictal discharges (*), confirmed on the real EEG.

5. Inactive, flat trace: mainly inactive (isoelectric tracing) background below 5 μV.

Correlation between amplitude-integrated electroencephalography and standard electroencephalography

Several studies have performed aEEG and standard EEG simultaneously to compare the two techniques. Overall, the aEEG and EEG background patterns in the sick full-term infant seemed to correlate [18,19]. Assessment of background pattern and the effect of hypoxia or hypotension have also been studied in different animal species, showing that electrocortical brain activity is more rapidly affected by hypotension than by hypoxia [20–22].

Prognostic value of amplitude-integrated electroencephalography background patterns

Over the years, several groups have studied the relationship between the background pattern recorded within 3 to 12 hours after birth and subsequent neurodevelopmental outcome [14–16,20,23–25]. The first studies assessed the aEEG during the first 12 to 24 hours, but because of recent interest in early intervention, studies have assessed aEEG as early as 3 to 6 hours after birth to see whether aEEG could play a role in identifying infants at risk for developing neonatal encephalopathy [13–15]. These studies assessed the predictive value of a poor background pattern (burst suppression, CLV, flat trace) for subsequent poor neurodevelopmental outcome,

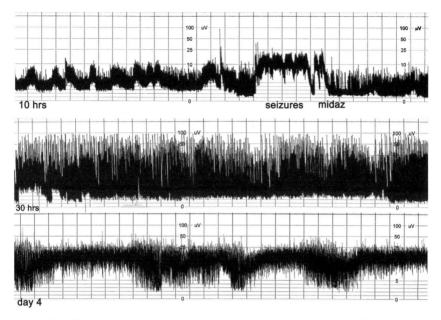

Fig. 3. The different background patterns during recovery over a 4-day period. The top recording shows low voltage with a rise during a period of 40 minutes of protracted seizure activity. After administration of midazolam, the recording briefly shows a flat trace. The middle part of the recording shows recovery to a burst suppression pattern. On day 4 a continuous voltage pattern has appeared with some rather irregular-looking sleep–wake cycling (Lectromed 5330, Olympic Medical, Seattle, Washington).

showing that the predictive values obtained by different groups were very similar (Table 1). Positive and negative predictive values were slightly lower when aEEG was assessed at 3 instead of 6 hours after birth, but they were still considered sufficiently high to use this technique for early selection in hypothermia or other intervention studies. A more recent study indicated that the sensitivity and specificity can be increased further when early aEEG evaluation is coupled with a clinical evaluation [25]. Compared with the neurologic examination performed within 12 hours after delivery, aEEG was more specific (89% vs. 78%) and had a higher positive predictive value (73% vs. 58%), but the best prediction of poor short-term outcome (14 of the 50 infants studied) was obtained when the results of the clinical and aEEG data were combined (94% and 85%, respectively).

Comparing aEEG with fractional cerebral tissue oxygen extraction (FTOE) measured using near-infrared spectroscopy showed that aEEG had predictive value within hours after birth, whereas FTOE was not significantly elevated in the children who had a poor outcome until 24 hours after birth [26].

We have recently reported on a small group of infants (18/161) that presented with a severely depressed aEEG background pattern within the first 6 hours after birth, but then recovered to a normal background pattern within

Table 1
Predictive value of a poor background pattern (burst suppression, continuous extremely low voltage, flat trace) for poor neurodevelopmental outcome in the neonatal period and infancy

Study	Time (h)	No. of patients	Sensitivity (%)	Specificity (%)	PPV (%)	NPV (%)
Hellström-Westas et al. [14]	6	47	95	89	86	96
Eken et al. [13]	6	34	94	79	84	92
Toet et al. [15]	6	68	91	86	86	96
Thornberg and Ekstrom-Jodal [23]	6	161	83	85	88	91
Toet et al. [15]	3	68	85	77	78	84

Abbreviations: NPV, negative predictive value; PPV, positive predictive value.

24 hours [27]. Early recovery of the background pattern was observed in only 6 of 65 (9%) infants who presented with a flat trace/CLV background pattern, but occurred in 12 of 24 (50%) infants with a burst suppression background pattern. Eleven of the 18 (61%) infants who showed a rapid recovery of the background pattern had a normal or mildly abnormal outcome, and 5 of these 11 initially had a flat trace/CLV background pattern. Although rapid recovery of the background pattern was more common in the burst suppression group, this finding was less often associated with a normal outcome. This difference in outcome for these two background pattern groups is of interest. The insult around the time of delivery in the flat trace/CLV group was almost invariably acute and severe, but presumably of shorter duration than in those who showed a persistent flat trace/CLV background pattern and those who showed a burst suppression pattern. aEEG alone was apparently not sufficient for an accurate prediction in the burst suppression group. We therefore performed additional neurophysiologic (visual- and somatosensory-evoked potentials) and neuroimaging studies (ultrasound and MRI) in this high-risk group. This study stressed the importance of continuing aEEG monitoring beyond the first 12 to 24 hours after birth.

Longer periods of monitoring also allow assessment of the presence, quality, and time of onset of sleep–wake cycling (SWC) (see Fig. 2). We have recently shown that these factors reflect the severity of the hypoxic-ischemic insult to which newborns have been exposed [28]. The time of SWC onset was shown to predict neurodevelopmental outcome based on whether the SWC returns before 36 hours (good outcome) or after 36 hours (bad outcome) (Fig. 4A). Using this method, accurate predictions were made in 82% of the 171 newborn infants who had differing degrees of encephalopathy, agreeing with two other recent reports [24,29]. Although infants treated with several antiepileptic drugs for seizures experienced a significantly later SWC onset, using one or two antiepileptic drugs did not have a significant effect on time of SWC onset (Fig. 4B).

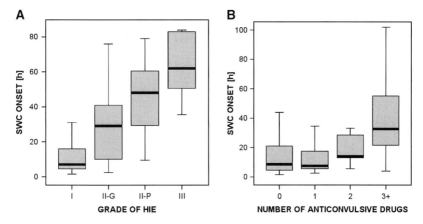

Fig. 4. (*A*) Relation between degree of hypoxic-ischemic encephalopathy and time of SWC onset in hours after birth. (*B*) Effect of number of antiepileptic drugs on time of SWC onset. (*Reproduced from* Osredkar D, Toet MC, van Rooij LGM, et al. Sleep-wake cycling on amplitude-integrated EEG in full-term newborns with hypoxic-ischemic encephalopathy. Pediatrics 2005;115(2):327–32; with permission).

Detection of epileptic seizure activity

A rapid rise of the lower and upper margins of the aEEG tracing suggests an ictal discharge (Fig. 5). Seizures can be recognized as single seizures, repetitive seizures, and status epilepticus. The latter usually has a "saw-tooth" pattern. Correct interpretation is greatly improved by simultaneous raw EEG recording available on the digital devices (Fig. 6). Increasing use of continuous monitoring has revealed that subclinical seizures are common and tend to be seen after the first antiepileptic drug is administered [2,3]. This so-called "uncoupling" or "electroclinical dissociation" was recently reported by several groups and found in 50% to 60% of the children studied [2,3]. The aEEG can play an important role in detecting these subclinical seizures. Awareness of this phenomenon has revealed the poor therapeutic effect of most of the commonly used antiepileptic drugs; drugs that were considered to have a good therapeutic effect mainly appear to suppress the clinical symptoms. Continuous EEG or aEEG recording, preferably with simultaneous video recording, is therefore required to assess the therapeutic effect of antiepileptic drugs.

A single-channel or even a two-channel EEG will not detect all seizures. Unsurprisingly, because of the nature of the technique, very brief seizure activity and focal seizure activity may be missed [19,30]. Infants who have focal seizures, however, tend to develop more widespread ictal discharges during continuous monitoring, which will be identified [19]. The long duration of aEEG monitoring therefore appears to outweigh the limitations of obtaining detailed information during a much shorter, 30-minute standard EEG. Whether the use of two or more channels is indicated in all at-risk

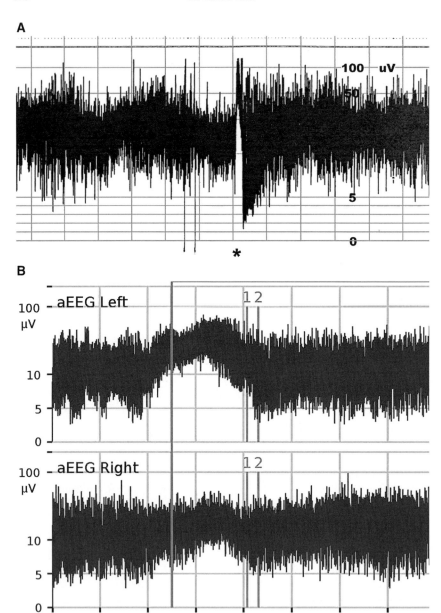

Fig. 5. Two recordings with an ictal discharge, confirmed with the simultaneous "real EEG"; The ictal discharge on the left (*A*) (Olympic 6000, Olympic Medical, Seattle, Washington) shows an abrupt rise of upper and lower margin and is of rather short duration with postictal suppression. The ictal discharge (*B*) on the right (BRM2, BrainZ, BrainZ Instruments, Auckland, New Zealand) is rather protracted and does not show an acute or sharp rise of lower and upper margin.

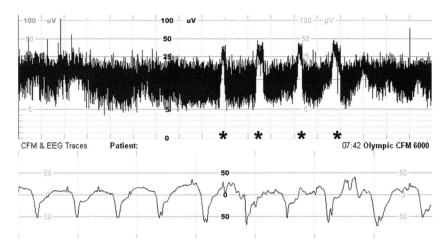

Fig. 6. Repetitive epileptic discharges on a CNV background pattern in a child who has a middle cerebral artery infarct; raw EEG indicated by the first asterisk, showing rhythmic activity.

infants is still debated. In our own population of full-term infants admitted with neonatal encephalopathy or seizures, 10% had a predominantly unilateral lesion (Fig. 7). Although some ictal discharges arose from the affected hemisphere, the discharge could usually be recognized on the cross-cerebral recording (Fig. 8).

The use of aEEG should not be restricted to full-term infants who have NE associated with problems around the time of delivery. Other conditions presenting with NE or seizures in the neonatal period, including meningoencephalitis, metabolic disorders, congenital malformations, use of muscle paralysis, post–open-heart surgery, and extracorporeal membrane oxygenation, are indications for this technique [31,32].

Summary

Experience with continuous aEEG is increasing and many NICUs would now find it hard to imagine treating a full-term infant who has NE without

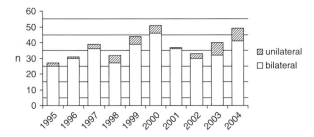

Fig. 7. Full-term infants admitted with NE or seizures (N = 389) between 1995 and 2004 with predominantly unilateral parenchymal lesions (n = 41, 10%).

A

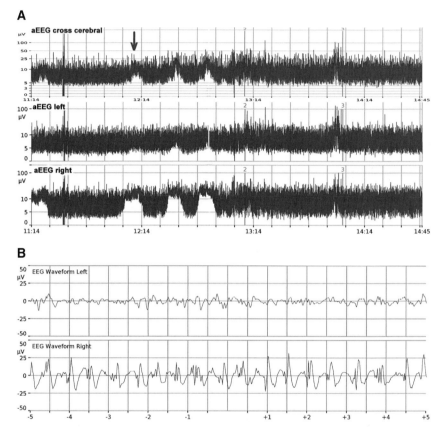

B

Fig. 8. (*A, B*) Full-term infant who has right-sided middle cerebral artery infarct, showing four right-sided discharges on the aEEG with confirmation on the raw EEG of the second one (*arrow*) (BRM2). The cross cerebral aEEG would not have identified the first discharge, but did identify the subsequent 3 discharges. The child developed a mild hemiplegia.

this equipment. The three main features an aEEG provides include (1) the background pattern, showing the activity at admission to the NICU and the rate of recovery during the first 24 to 48 hours after birth; (2) the presence or absence of SWC; and (3) the presence of electrographic seizure discharges. Access to the real EEG on the new digital machines has enabled better reading of aEEGs, especially for electrographic discharges. New software has become available that enables experts to calculate the interburst interval and number of bursts per hour online, which have been shown to have predictive value using the standard EEG [12]. Interpretation of the different background patterns has also become more reliable using the new "insight" gray scale (Fig. 9). However, the aEEG is a monitoring device and does not replace a standard EEG. Especially in the more intermediate discontinuous background pattern, correct interpretation, and particularly identification of ictal discharges, may be difficult. Most centers, therefore,

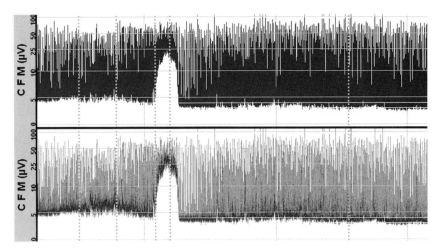

Fig. 9. An ictal discharge on a burst suppression pattern. This background pattern is best recognized and the sharp rise of the lower margin is better appreciated with the "insight" gray scale (Olympic 6000, Olympic Medical, Seattle, Washington).

will experience an increased number of standard EEG requests rather than a decrease. With some of the digital aEEG machines, connection to a network and online access to the neurophysiology department may be possible, even from home.

As the use of aEEG has increased, experts have become more aware of the limited effects of commonly used antiepileptic drugs such as phenobarbitone and phenytoin [1], and other second-line antiepileptic drugs, including lidocaine and midazolam [33–36]. Whether treating electrographic discharges is in the best interest of the infant is uncertain. Two groups of infants treated for clinical and subclinical seizures showed a lower incidence of postneonatal epilepsy (8%–9%) compared with those who underwent treatment only for EEG-confirmed clinical seizures [37–40], suggesting that treatment of clinical and subclinical seizures has a potential benefit. Data from other groups supported this finding [41,42]. The first randomized study of treatment of subclinical seizures (SuSeQ) is underway, with 11 neonatal units participating in the Netherlands and Belgium.

Data obtained in animal experiments suggested a possible apoptotic neurodegenerative effect of commonly used antiepileptic drugs at concentrations relevant for seizure control in humans [43]. New drugs such as lamotrigine, which also has a neuroprotective effect, will probably be studied in the near future. Dzhala and colleagues [44,45] recently described other mechanisms in a neonatal rat experiment, shedding new light on treatment of neonatal seizures. They illustrated that the Na^{+}-K^{+}-$2Cl^{-}$ cotransporter (NKCC1) facilitates the accumulation of Cl^{-} in neurons and facilitates seizures in the developing brain, whereas bumetanide blocked NKCC1 and therefore should be useful in treating neonatal seizures.

In conclusion, experts have become increasingly aware of the importance of continuous monitoring of electrocortical activity. Although aEEG may provide limited information regarding seizure detection, it is reliable in recognizing background abnormalities, which have been shown to be strongly predictive of neurodevelopmental outcome. Every child now admitted to a NICU with NE or seizures should be placed on a continuous monitor, whether it is an aEEG or, ideally, a multichannel video-EEG attached to a hospital network.

Acknowledgments

We are especially grateful to Kees van Huffelen and Mireille Bourez from the Department of Neurophysiology for good collaboration and continuous support in the work with aEEG.

References

[1] Painter MJ, Scher MS, Stein AD, et al. Phenobarbital compared with Phenytoin for the treatment of neonatal seizures. N Engl J Med 1999;341(7):485–9.

[2] Boylan GB, Rennie JM, Pressler RM, et al. Phenobarbitone, neonatal seizures, and video-EEG. Arch Dis Child Fetal Neonatal Ed 2002;86(3):F165–70.

[3] Scher MS, Alvin J, Gaus L, et al. Uncoupling of EEG-clinical neonatal seizures after antiepileptic drug use. Pediatr Neurol 2003;28(4):277–80.

[4] Maynard DE. EEG analysis using an analogue frequency analyser and a digital computer. Electroencephalogr Clin Neurophysiol 1967;23(5):487.

[5] Prior PF. EEG monitoring and evoked potentials in brain ischaemia. Br J Anaesth 1985; 57(1):63–81.

[6] Prior PF, Maynard DE. Monitoring cerebral function. Long-term recordings of cerebral electrical activity and evoked potentials. Amsterdam: Elsevier; 1986.

[7] Bjerre I, Hellström-Westas L, Rosen I, et al. Monitoring of cerebral function after severe birth asphyxia in infancy. Arch Dis Child 1983;58(12):997–1002.

[8] Verma UL, Archbald F, Tejani NA, et al. Cerebral function monitor in the neonate. I: normal patterns. Dev Med Child Neurol 1984;26(2):154–61.

[9] Hellström-Westas L, Rosen I, Svenningsen NW. Silent seizures in sick infants in early life. Acta Paediatr Scand 1985;74(5):741–8.

[10] Gluckman PD, Wyatt JS, Azzopardi D, et al. Selective head cooling with mild systemic hypothermia after neonatal encephalopathy: multicentre randomised trial. Lancet 2005; 365(9460):663–70.

[11] Holmes GL, Lombroso CT. Prognostic value of background patterns in the neonatal EEG. J Clin Neurophysiol 1993;10(3):323–52.

[12] Menache CC, Bourgeois BF, Volpe JJ. Prognostic value of neonatal discontinuous. Pediatr Neurol 2002;27(2):93–101.

[13] Eken P, Toet MC, Groenendaal F, et al. Predictive value of early neuroimaging, pulsed Doppler and neurophysiology in full term infants with hypoxic-ischemic encephalopathy. Arch Dis Child Fetal Neonatal Ed 1995;73(2):F75–80.

[14] Hellström-Westas L, Rosen I, Svenningsen NW. Predictive value of early continuous amplitude integrated EEG recordings on outcome after severe birth asphyxia in full term infants. Arch Dis Child Fetal Neonatal Ed 1995;72(2):F34–8.

[15] Toet MC, Hellström-Westas L, Groenendaal F, et al. Amplitude integrated EEG 3 and 6 hours after birth in full term neonates with hypoxic-ischaemic encephalopathy. Arch Dis Child Fetal Neonatal Ed 1999;81(1):F19–23.

[16] Al Naqeeb N, Edwards AD, Cowan F, et al. Assessment of neonatal encephalopathy by amplitude integrated electroencephalography. Pediatrics 1999;103(6 Pt 1):1263–71.

[17] Hellström-Westas L, Rosén I, de Vries LS, et al. Amplitude-integrated EEG classification and interpretation in preterm and term infants. Neonatal Review 2006;7(2):e76–86.

[18] Hellström-Westas L. Comparison between tape-recorded and amplitude integrated EEG monitoring sick newborn infants. Acta Paediatr Scand 1992;81(10):812–9.

[19] Toet MC, van der Meij W, de Vries LS, et al. Comparison between simultaneously recorded amplitude integrated EEG (Cerebral Function Monitor) and standard EEG in neonates-Pediatrics 2002;109(5):772–9.

[20] Bunt JE, Gavilanes AW, Reulen JP, et al. The influence of acute hypoxemia and hypovolemic hypotension of neuronal brain activity measured by the cerebral function monitor in newborn piglets. Neuropediatrics 1996;27(5):260–4.

[21] Gavilanes AW, Vles JS, von Siebenthal K, et al. Electrocortical brain activity, cerebral haemodynamics and oxygenation during progressive hypotension in newborn piglets. Clin Neurophysiol 2001;112(1):52–9.

[22] Van Os S, Klaessens J, Hopman J, et al. Preservation of electrocortical brain activity during hypoxemia in preterm lambs. Exp Brain Res 2003;151(1):54–9.

[23] Thornberg E, Ekstrom-Jodal B. Cerebral function monitoring: a method of predicting outcome in term neonates after severe perinatal asphyxia. Acta Paediatr 1994;83(6):596–601.

[24] Ter Horst HJ, Sommer C, Bergman KA, et al. Prognostic significance of amplitude-integrated EEG during the first 72 hours after birth in severely asphyxiated neonates. Pediatr Res 2004;55(6):1026–33.

[25] Shalak LF, Laptook AR, Velaphi SC, et al. Amplitude-integrated electroencephalography coupled with an early neurologic examination enhances prediction of term infants at risk for persistent encephalopathy. Pediatrics 2003;111(2):351–7.

[26] Toet MC, Lemmers PM, van Schelven LJ, et al. Cerebral oxygenation and electrical activity after birth asphyxia: their relation to outcome. Pediatrics 2006;117(2):333–9.

[27] van Rooij LG, Toet MC, Osredkar D, et al. Recovery of amplitude integrated electroencephalographic background patterns within 24 hours of perinatal asphyxia. Arch Dis Child Fetal Neonatal Ed 2005;90(3):F245–51.

[28] Osredkar D, Toet MC, van Rooij LGM, et al. Sleep-wake cycling on amplitude-integrated EEG in full-term newborns with hypoxic-ischemic encephalopathy. Pediatrics 2005;115(2):327–32.

[29] Thorngren-Jerneck K, Hellström-Westas L, Ryding E, et al. Cerebral glucose metabolism and early EEG/aEEG in term newborn infants with hypoxic-ischemic encephalopathy. Pediatr Res 2003;54(6):854–60.

[30] Rennie JM, Chorley G, Boylan GB, et al. Non-expert use of the cerebral function monitor for neonatal seizure detection. Arch Dis Child Fetal Neonatal Ed 2004;89(1):F37–40.

[31] Toet MC, Flinterman A, Laar I, et al. Cerebral oxygen saturation and electrical brain activity before, during, and up to 36 hours after arterial switch procedure in neonates without pre-existing brain damage: its relationship to neurodevelopmental outcome. Exp Brain Res 2005;165(3):343–50.

[32] Pappas A, Shankaran S, Stockmann PT, et al. Changes in amplitude-integrated electroencephalography in neonates treated with extracorporeal membrane oxygenation: a pilot study. J Pediatr 2006;148(1):125–7.

[33] Boylan GB, Rennie JM, Chorley G, et al. Second-line anticonvulsant treatment of neonatal seizures. Neurology 2004;62(3):486–8.

[34] Hellström-Westas L, Svenningsen NW, Westgren U, et al. Lidocaine for treatment of severe seizures in newborn infants. II. Blood concentrations of lidocaine and metabolites during intravenous infusion. Acta Paediatr 1992;81(10):35–9.

[35] Malingre M, Van Rooij LGM, Rademaker CMA, et al. Development of an optimal lido-
     caine infusion strategy in neonatal seizures. Eur J Pediatr, in press.
[36] van Leuven K, Groenendaal F, Toet MC, et al. Midazolam and amplitude integrated EEG in
     asphyxiated full-term neonates. Acta Paediatr 2004;93(9):1221-7.
[37] Hellström-Westas L, Blennow G, Lindroth M, et al. Low risk of seizure recurrence after
     early withdrawal of anti-epileptic treatment in the neonatal period. Arch Dis Child 1995;
     72(1):F97-101.
[38] Toet MC, Groenendaal F, Osredkar D, et al. Postneonatal epilepsy following amplitude-
     integrated EEG-detected neonatal seizures. Pediatr Neurol 2005;32(4):241-7.
[39] Clancy RR, Legido A. Postnatal epilepsy after EEG-confirmed neonatal seizures. Epilepsia
     1991;32(1):69-76.
[40] Brunquell PJ, Glennon CS, Dimario FJ, et al. Prediction of outcome based on clinical seizure
     type in newborn infants. J Pediatr 2002;140(6):707-12.
[41] Miller SP, Weiss J, Barnwell A, et al. Seizure-associated brain injury in term newborns with
     perinatal asphyxia. Neurology 2002;58(4):542-8.
[42] Oliveira AJ, Nunes M, Haertel LM, et al. Duration of rhythmic EEG patterns in neonates:
     new evidence for clinical and prognostic significance of brief rhythmic discharges. Clin
     Neurophysiol 2000;111(9):1646-53.
[43] Bittigau P, Sifringer M, Genz K, et al. Antiepileptic drugs and apoptosis in the developing
     brain. Proc Natl Acad Sci USA 2002;99(23):15089-94.
[44] Dzhala VI, Talos DM, Sdrulla DA, et al. NKCC1 transporter facilitates seizures in the
     developing brain. Nat Med 2005;11(11):1205-13.
[45] Fukuda A. Diuretic soothes seizures in newborns. Nat Med 2005;11(11):1153-4.

ELSEVIER
SAUNDERS

CLINICS IN
PERINATOLOGY

Clin Perinatol 33 (2006) 633–647

Continuous Electroencephalography Monitoring of the Preterm Infant

Lena Hellström-Westas, MD, PhD

Neonatal Intensive Care Unit, Department of Pediatrics, Lund University Hospital,
SE-22185 Lund, Sweden

The rationale for using continuous electroencephalography (EEG) in newborn infants is to obtain information on brain function in sick term or preterm infants who may be incapable of showing symptoms of compromised brain activity. Continuous monitoring of electrocortical activity includes evaluation of overall background activity, detection of subclinical seizure activity, and verification of clinically suspected seizures. Continuous EEG monitoring has been used increasingly in neonatal intensive care units (NICU) because studies have shown that a trend measure of the EEG, the amplitude-integrated EEG (aEEG), is sensitive for very early prediction of outcome in term asphyxiated infants [1,2]. The aEEG is also increasingly being used in preterm infants, as seen in several recent studies [3–9]. Although the value of continuous EEG monitoring in preterm infants with brain injury has not been proven, some studies have shown that development of intraventricular hemorrhage (IVH) and white matter injury (WMI) is associated with early changes in the EEG as evaluated by aEEG and spectral edge frequency, which is another trend measure of the EEG [10–12].

This article shows how the aEEG can be used in preterm infants as a clinical tool in the NICU, focusing on aEEG because this method for continuous EEG monitoring is used most in preterm infants. Experience with EEG monitoring is rapidly increasing and future studies may prove that other trends or combinations of trends, depending on the indication for monitoring, may provide similar or more accurate information.

During the neonatal period, preterm infants may be exposed to several unpleasant or stressful stimuli that may affect long-term outcome [13,14]. EEG monitoring systems suitable for preterm infants should therefore

This work was supported by Grant No 0037 from the Swedish Medical Research Council, and by a Grant (ALF-LUA) from the Medical Faculty at Lund University.

E-mail address: lena.hellstrom-westas@med.lu.se

add as little stress or discomfort as possible. A main concern is the electrodes that are used, which should be simple to apply because cumbersome application of electrodes, reapplication if they come loose, or pressure/pain on the head from electrodes may add to the overall burden of noxious stimuli in these infants.

The normal amplitude-integrated electroencephalography in preterm infants

Some basic knowledge about the standard EEG is a prerequisite for using EEG monitoring. The clinical interpretation of EEG and aEEG is based on pattern recognition. The normal EEG background of the extremely preterm infant is discontinuous, characterized by periods with high voltage activity (burst) interspersed with periods of low amplitude (interburst interval), and is called *tracé discontinu* (Fig. 1). With increasing maturation, the EEG background becomes gradually more continuous and includes shorter interburst intervals, longer duration of bursts, and higher amplitude during the low-amplitude activity. Very preterm infants may also have periods of continuous EEG activity, but these are usually not as sustained as in the term infant. Published data for normal maturational changes in the EEG include quantified values for degree of continuity during sleep and wakefulness, and distribution and topographic evolution of activity over the cerebral hemispheres [15–21].

Intensive care treatment, illness, and medications could affect the EEG background, and therefore describing what constitutes a normal EEG in the extremely preterm infant has been a problem. A few small studies describe the early EEG in extremely preterm infants who were presumed healthy and underwent normal long-term follow-up [18–20]. Of special relevance for clinical EEG monitoring of preterm infants are data on normal interburst intervals at different gestational ages. Recently published

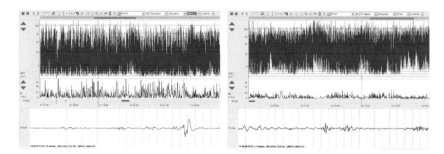

Fig. 1. Six-hour aEEG and interburst interval (below aEEG) recordings from the first day of life in two stable preterm infants, the left from an infant born at 23 weeks' gestation, and the right from an infant at 28 weeks' gestation. Twenty-five seconds of EEG, corresponding with the gray vertical line in the aEEG, is displayed below. The EEG shows a discontinuous pattern called *tracé discontinu*, the more mature infant showing more variability and shorter interburst intervals.

EEG data indicate that interburst intervals should ideally be shorter than 30 seconds and should not exceed 45 seconds even in the most immature infants [18–20,22]. A few studies of preterm infants using EEG/aEEG have indicated that electrocortical background activity was more discontinuous during the first days of life and became more continuous during subsequent days [8,10,21]. No explanation is currently available for this finding, which could be caused by postnatal depression and recovery after delivery, or an effect of arousal and adaptation to extrauterine life. Two recent studies also show that maturation of aEEG continuity measures seem to be somewhat accelerated during the first weeks of life in preterm infants [7,9].

The first studies that presented aEEG data from normal newborn infants were performed in the late 1970s and the 1980s [23–25]. These studies included stable, moderately preterm infants aged primarily between 30 and 31 weeks' gestation, but only a few of the extremely preterm infants that now inhabit the NICU [10,11]. Later studies further described and quantified aEEG tracings, especially in extremely preterm infants [5–7,9]. Cyclicity of the aEEG pattern, indicative of sleep–wake cycling (SWC), can be seen at approximately 25 to 26 gestational weeks in infants who have no IVH. aEEG development during maturation can be described as an ongoing changing pattern that becomes increasingly continuous with progressively better-developed SWC. The aEEG pattern can also be quantified in different ways, such as percentage of activity over a certain amplitude or interburst interval. Viniker and colleagues [23] showed that gestational age and the amplitude of the lower border of the aEEG during the discontinuous period (ie, quiet sleep) had a linear correlation. A similar observation was later made in more preterm infants [5]. Table 1 summarizes normal aEEG features in preterm infants at different gestational ages [26]. High-frequency ventilation may disturb the aEEG recording. Although the general background pattern and interburst interval may still be possible to evaluate (although more uncertain), comparisons with normative data for aEEG-continuity may become impossible, as shown in Fig. 2.

Sleep–wake states

Standard criteria for assessing sleep–wake states include evaluation of respiration, cardiac activity, movements, and rapid eye movements. In the aEEG, SWC appears as a sinusoidal pattern with varying bandwidth and continuity [4,5,25]. The aEEG is more discontinuous during quiet sleep than during wakefulness and active sleep, and is represented by a broader tracing with lower minimum amplitude. The average duration of quiet sleep periods is 24 to 28 minutes between 32 and 36 postconceptional weeks, and slightly longer at night, but otherwise relatively stable and not affected by incubator covers or developmental care intervention [27,28]. The aEEG

Table 1
Summary of normal findings in the early amplitude-integrated electroencephalography in relation to gestational age in preterm infants

Gestational or postconceptional age (wk)	Dominating background pattern	Sleep–wake cycling	Minimum amplitude (μV)	Maximum amplitude (μV)	Burst/h
24–25	DC	(+)	2–5	25–50 (−100)	>100
26–27	DC	(+)	2–5	25–50 (−100)	>100
28–29	DC/(C)	(+)/+	2–5	25–30	>100
30–31	C/(DC)	+	2–6	20–30	>100
32–33	C/DC in QS	+	2–6	20–30	>100
34–35	C/DC in QS	+	3–7	15–25	>100
36–37	C/DC in QS	+	4–8	17–35	>100
38+	C/DC in QS	+	7–8	15–25	>100

Abbreviations: C, continuous activity; C/(DC), mainly continuous activity, some discontinuous activity; C/DC in QS, continuous activity, discontinuous in quiet sleep; DC, discontinuous activity; DC/(C), mainly discontinuous activity, some continuous activity; SWC +, developed SWC; SWC (+), immature SWC.

From Hellström-Westas L, Rosén I, De Vries LS, et al. Amplitude-integrated EEG: classification and interpretation in preterm and term infants. Neoreviews 2006;7:e76–87.

patterns representing active sleep and wakefulness cannot be distinguished. Transitional sleep is often evaluated in neonatal sleep studies, and periods of transitional sleep can be seen in the aEEG just before and immediately after quiet sleep periods, although this measure has not been specifically evaluated. The correspondence between aEEG pattern and clinical criteria for sleep–wake states (awake, quiet sleep, and active sleep) has been evaluated in preterm infants born at 29 to 34 weeks' gestation [29]. SWC in the aEEG is clearly discernible in stable infants from approximately 30 weeks' gestation [7,25,29]. Most extremely immature infants have SWC, although not as well defined or organized as more mature preterm infants [30]. In the aEEG, immature SWC may appear as sinusoidal changes of the

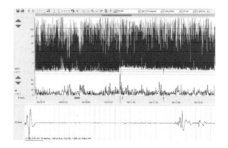

Fig. 2. Moderate increase in aEEG baseline amplitude when high-frequency oscillatory ventilation was started, but no change in interburst interval or general background pattern.

minimum amplitude, usually with a rather short duration of approximately 30 to 60 minutes (see Fig. 1) [4,7,11].

Intraventricular hemorrhage, white matter injury, and electroencephalography/amplitude-integrated electroencephalography

The EEG undergoes characteristic but nonspecific changes when IVH and WMI develop in preterm infants [31–34]. Studies in the 1980s showed that the degree of early EEG abnormality correlated with neurologic outcome and the extent of IVH [31,32]. Furthermore, in preterm infants dying with IVH, the number of damaged brain structures correlated even better with EEG abnormality than with the degree of IVH [35]. Studies using continuous EEG monitoring during the first days of life showed that development of IVH and cerebral echodensities was associated with early amplitude depression and the presence of epileptic seizures, mainly subclinical (Fig. 3) [10,11,33,34]. The initial amplitude depression correlated with the degree of IVH and with outcome in infants born extremely preterm (Table 2) [11]. Recovery of electrocortical background activity occurred after a few days, but was delayed in infants who had higher degrees of IVH, as seen in Fig. 4 [10]. The rate of aEEG recovery during the first days of life in surviving infants with grade 3 to 4 IVH was predictive of neurologic outcome [3]. Because the predominant normal EEG/aEEG in very preterm infants is discontinuous, early pattern recognition for prediction of outcome could not be used as it was in the term asphyxiated infant. Instead, a measure of continuity was used, the *burst rate*, defined as the number of EEG bursts produced per hour. In surviving infants, the maximum number of bursts per hour during the first 24 to 48 hours of life differed among those who had "fair" and those who had "poor" outcome (median 156, range 103–179 vs. median 102, range 73–156, respectively; $P = .002$). At the same interval,

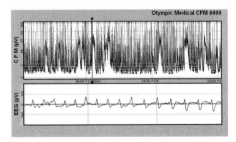

Fig. 3. A 3-hour aEEG from the second day of life in a preterm infant born at 25 weeks' gestation who developed a unilateral IVH grade 4. The aEEG shows at least 10 subclinical seizures, each with duration of 5 to 10 minutes. The seizure activity in the aEEG is characterized by an abrupt rise in amplitude. The EEG from the fifth seizure (*dashed vertical line*) is displayed below the aEEG trace.

Table 2
Percentage of activity above 3 μV (% continuity) during the first 72 hours of life in 25 extremely
preterm infants (gestational age ≤ 27 weeks, mean 25.7) in relation to degree of intraventricular
hemorrhage and outcome at 2 years of age

	% continuity in aEEG	Outcome at 2-year follow-up
No IVH (n = 7)	39.8	All normal
IVH grade 1–2 (n = 8)	28.3	5 normal, 1 handicap, 2 died
IVH grade 3–4 (n = 10)	8.5	4 handicap, 6 died

Data from Hellström-Westas L, Rosen I, Svenningsen NW. Cerebral function monitoring
during the first week of life in extremely small low birthweight (ESLBW) infants. Neuropediatrics 1991;22(1):27–32.

maximum bursts per hour less than 130 had a sensitivity of 70%, specificity of 92%, positive predictive value of 95%, and negative predictive value of 60% for predicting death or survival in infants who had "poor" outcome. Altogether 78% were correctly predicted [3]. The minimum number of bursts per hour was also measured, but was not associated with outcome, probably because this measure may be affected and lowered by several medications. Presence of SWC during the first 5 days of life was also associated with better outcome, but epileptic seizure activity was not associated with neurologic prognosis.

According to Watanabe and colleagues [36], EEG abnormalities in newborn infants can be classified as acute-stage or chronic-stage changes. The acute-stage EEG abnormalities occur during and shortly after the insult, and include amplitude depression, increased discontinuity, and presence of epileptic seizure activity. The chronic-stage changes develop over several weeks and may include disorganized or dysmature (ie, maturational delay of more than 2 weeks) background patterns [37,38]. Positive rolandic sharp waves (PRSWs) are markers of WMI that may emerge during this stage. The number of PRSWs appearing in the EEG has been associated with the risk for developing cerebral palsy [39]. The aEEG is sensitive for detecting acute-stage changes in the EEG, but can probably not be used to evaluate chronic changes. Although the minimum amplitude of the aEEG (lower border of the aEEG) and gestational age seem to correlate, no studies have assessed whether this feature can be used to evaluate maturational delay in preterm infants. However, although the aEEG is a superb method for clinical long-term monitoring in the NICU, it cannot provide detailed information and should be regarded as a complement to the standard EEG.

Effects of medications on electroencephalography/amplitude-integrated electroencephalography

Several medications may affect the EEG and aEEG of preterm infants. The general response is a transient depression of background activity that

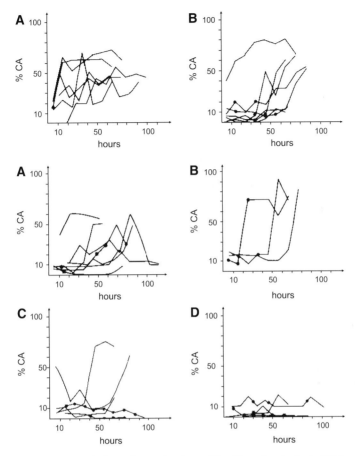

Fig. 4. Thirty-two preterm infants of gestational ages 25 to 32 weeks who had aEEG recordings started within 24 hours after birth and with at least 50 hours duration. The average percentage of continuous activity above 3 μV was calculated for each 10-hour interval and displayed in relation to degree of IVH for each infant. Asterisks denote periods with seizure activity. The upper two figures show infants who have no IVH: (*A*) infants who have normal serum calcium and (*B*) infants who have hypocalcemia. The four lower figures show infants who developed IVH: (*A*) grade 1, (*B*) grade 2, (*C*) grade 3, and (*D*) grade 4. (*From* Greisen G, Hellstrom-Westas L, Lou H, et al. EEG depression and germinal layer hemorrhage in the newborn. Acta Paediatr Scand 1987;76(3):519–25; with permission.)

can be seen as either a decrease in burst rate (increased interburst intervals) or a general depression of amplitude. The duration of the EEG response varies from minutes (with surfactant, morphine, and diazepam) to hours (with morphine, sufentanil, and phenobarbital) (Figs. 5 and 6). Consequently, possible effects from previous medications must be considered when interpreting aEEG tracings [40–43]. Administering sufentanil was shown to induce loss of SWC in the EEG, which is also likely to occur after

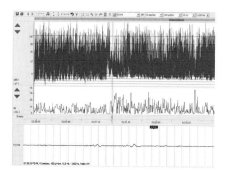

Fig. 5. A 2-hour recording of aEEG and interburst interval from an infant born at 24 gestational weeks. The infant was on high-frequency oscillatory ventilation, which can be seen as low-amplitude fast rhythmic changes in the EEG trace (25 seconds displayed below the other traces). The infant did not develop IVH or periventricular leukomalacia and the burst density in the aEEG is good. After administration of surfactant (*vertical gray line*), a decrease in burst rate can be seen in the aEEG, which is also reflected by an increase in interburst interval (trend below the aEEG).

administration of other opioids or sedative medications, but this feature has not been evaluated in other studies [43].

Effects of blood pressure, persistent ductus arteriosus, and carbon dioxide on electroencephalography/amplitude-integrated electroencephalography

In preterm infants who require intensive care treatment, several conditions occur that may affect electrocortical activity. Arterial hypotension may affect EEG activity if severe enough to decrease cerebral blood flow (CBF) and neuronal activity. Electrocortical activity in preterm infants seems to be preserved at very low CBF, as measured with aEEG and xenon

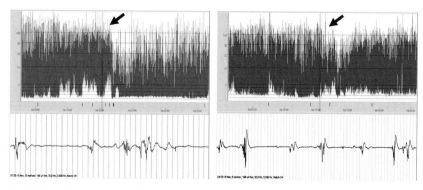

Fig. 6. Recording from two infants born at 26 weeks' gestation. Both recordings show transient decreases in cerebral activity, caused by a pneumothorax in the left recording and after administration of diazepam in the right recording, as shown by the arrows.

133 clearance [44]. However, the lowest CBF measurements, down to 5 mL/ 100g/min, were related to discontinuous aEEG activity and severe intracranial hemorrhagic or ischemic morbidity. In hypotensive preterm infants, volume administration immediately increased the aEEG burst rate in 5 of 12 preterm infants, but the aEEG recovery was slower and not as distinct in the other infants [45]. Recent studies support earlier findings on the relationship between EEG and blood flow, showing a correlation with early low cardiac output and lower EEG continuity [46]. Small changes in aEEG amplitude during blood exchange transfusion seemed to be related to changes in mean arterial blood pressure [47]. However, moderately decreased CBF velocity in infants who have a persistent patent ductus arteriosus but no intracranial abnormality does not seem to affect EEG activity [48]. Carbon dioxide levels and acidosis may also affect EEG background in preterm infants, and severe hypercarbia and hypocarbia seem to decrease continuity and burst rate [49,50].

Case reports have shown transient aEEG deterioration of cerebral activity in preterm infants during severe hypoglycemia and development of pneumothorax [51]. However, no aEEG changes were shown in moderately hypoglycemic term infants born to mothers who had diabetes [52]. A reason for the lack of aEEG changes is probably that this method is too crude to detect possible subtle electrocortical changes during moderate hypoglycemia. The preserved aEEG background could also be explained by the ability of the neonatal brain to respond to metabolic demands during hypoglycemia through the use of alternate substrates and compensatory increases in CBF [53]. No other clinical studies have evaluated continuous EEG during neonatal hypoglycemia.

The reversibility and recovery of the electrocortical background changes in preterm infants affected by low cardiac output or severe hypotension are probably related to the severity and duration of the condition. The cerebral response may also be related to prior hypoxic-ischemic insults, such as birth asphyxia. Brief deterioration in cerebral substrate delivery caused by acute changes in blood flow or oxygenation is more likely to result in full recovery, whereas more long-standing conditions that affect cerebral function may show poor reversibility of the EEG.

Evaluation of amplitude-integrated electroencephalography during neonatal intensive care

What type of aEEG abnormalities could one expect to find that might have clinical relevance and implications for the care of preterm infants? Current knowledge about aEEG in preterm infants is limited. No data currently show that early and accurate prediction of later outcome is possible in preterm infants, although results from some studies indicate that early EEG abnormalities are present in infants who develop IVH and WMI [3,10–12].

Furthermore, no data indicate that such information, if available, could lead to specific interventions that parallel the term postasphyxial situation [54]. However, information obtained from continuous EEG monitoring in preterm infants can still be used to direct medical investigations and treatment, and can also be used to counsel parents. Indications for EEG monitoring in preterm infants are similar to those for term infants, including

1. Monitoring cerebral function and recovery during intensive care treatment (see Figs. 3 and 6; Fig. 7)
2. Detecting subclinical seizures or verifying epileptic seizure activity in infants who have subtle or nonspecific symptoms (Fig. 8)
3. Monitoring effects of antiepileptic treatment

Practical aspects

Different types of electrodes can be used. Single-use thin-needle subcutaneous electrodes are easy to apply after gentle skin disinfection, but may require adhesives. These electrodes are the quickest to apply during intensive care, and usually give excellent recordings with low impedance. A key question, however, is whether needle electrodes cause pain. Sometimes applying needle electrodes does not seem to affect the infant at all, but occasionally infants grimace briefly. Needle electrodes can probably be painful if they are pulled or dislocated during care procedures. Stick-on gel electrodes and standard silver-silverchloride cup electrodes also work well, but although their application does not include a skin-breaking procedure, the scrubbing required to prepare the skin and reapply electrodes could be uncomfortable.

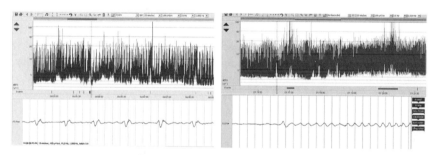

Fig. 7. Recordings from an infant who was severely asphyxiated, born after placental abruption at 33 weeks' gestation. The infant developed pulmonary hypertension and was supported by high-frequency ventilation and inhaled nitric oxide. The left tracing was obtained during the first day of life and shows a severely depressed pattern with mainly subclinical status epilepticus ("saw-tooth" pattern). The EEG shows slow rhythmic sharp-wave activity at the end of an electroclinical seizure (marked by a gray vertical line in the aEEG). The right tracing was recorded on the second day of life and shows a change in the aEEG background from burst suppression (*left*) to more continuous activity. The EEG shows the beginning of a subclinical seizure, corresponding with the gray vertical line in the aEEG.

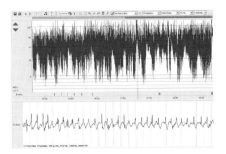

Fig. 8. Recordings from a preterm infant, born at 32 weeks' gestation, who had an initial uneventful course but developed viral meningitis at 4 weeks of age. The infant had no clinical seizures but was very irritable. The 3.5-hour recording shows a "saw-tooth" pattern representing recurrent seizures on a continuous aEEG background. Below the aEEG are 25 seconds of EEG representing the seizure, marked by a gray vertical line.

The bilateral parietal position (P3–P4 position, according to the international 10–20 system) is recommended for single-channel aEEG electrodes. This position was originally recommended for adults when recording with the first aEEG monitor, the cerebral function monitor, and was considered the most sensitive position for detecting adverse EEG changes caused by vascular compromise in watershed areas. When using a limited number of electrodes, some seizures will pass undetected. The risk for missing a seizure is reduced when more channels are used, but the complexity of the monitoring is also increased. For standard clinical monitoring, two-channel recordings with bilateral leads, such as frontoparietal, will probably become the preferred method. In all infants who have suspected seizure activity, a standard EEG should be recorded and indications for further evaluation by video-EEG monitoring considered.

Summary

Continuous EEG monitoring provides clinically relevant information even in the most preterm infants. Although early aEEG may detect preterm brain injury, it will probably not have the same high predictive sensitivity as in term asphyxiated infants. Development of brain injury in the extremely preterm infant is associated with acute hypoxic-ischemic insults, but is also affected by other factors such as perinatal inflammation, late onset sepsis, bronchopulmonary dysplasia, and postnatal nutrition [55–57].

The main indication for using aEEG and other continuous EEG trends in preterm infants is clinical surveillance, with the possibility of gaining additional relevant information that could be beneficial for a sick infant. EEG trends should be evaluated continuously during clinical monitoring. For practical clinical monitoring in the NICU, the aEEG can be compared with the continuously monitored single-channel ECG, whereas the full

ECG (and EEG) is recorded when additional and more detailed information is needed. The nonexpert interpretation and reduced number of EEG channels are limitations that users must be aware of when using the technique. It is well-known that antiepileptic treatment may extinguish clinical seizures while electrographic seizure activity persists [57]. Because of the limited number of electrodes in the aEEG, focal seizures may pass unrecognized [58].

In the most preterm infants, the best continuity or activity measure is probably the interburst interval. Increased discontinuity (increased interburst interval) and amplitude depression may signal clinical deterioration affecting the brain, but can also be seen in response to some medications. The continuous information on brain function obtained from an aEEG that is recorded for hours or days will probably contribute to an increased knowledge and understanding of the mechanisms for preterm brain injury and improved care. Future perspectives also include development of specific interventions to reduce hypoxic-ischemic brain injury in the preterm infant. Consequently, further investigation of the sensitivity of early continuous EEG is needed, especially in moderately preterm infants.

References

[1] Hellstrom-Westas L, Rosen I, Svenningsen NW. Predictive value of early continuous amplitude integrated EEG recordings on outcome after severe birth asphyxia in full term infants. Arch Dis Child Fetal Neonatal Ed 1995;72(1):F34–8.

[2] Eken P, Toet MC, Groenendaal F, et al. Predictive value of early neuroimaging, pulsed Doppler and neurophysiology in full term infants with hypoxic-ischaemic encephalopathy. Arch Dis Child Fetal Neonatal Ed 1995;73(2):F75–80.

[3] Hellström-Westas L, Klette H, Thorngren-Jerneck K, et al. Early prediction of outcome with aEEG in premature infants with large intraventricular haemorrhages. Neuropediatrics 2001; 32(6):319–24.

[4] Kuhle S, Klebermass K, Olischar M, et al. Sleep-wake cycles in preterm infants below 30 weeks of gestational age. Preliminary results of a prospective amplitude-integrated EEG study. Wien Klin Wochenschr 2001;113(7):219–23.

[5] Burdjalov VF, Baumgart S, Spitzer AR. Cerebral function monitoring: a new scoring system for the evaluation of brain maturation in neonates. Pediatrics 2003;112(4):855–61.

[6] Olischar M, Klebermass K, Kuhle S, et al. Reference values for amplitude-integrated electroencephalographic activity in preterm infants younger than 30 weeks' gestational age. Pediatrics 2004;113(1 Pt 1):e61–6.

[7] Sisman J, Campbell DE, Brion LP. Amplitude-integrated EEG in preterm infants: maturation of background pattern and amplitude voltage with postmenstrual age and gestational age. J Perinatol 2005;25(6):391–6.

[8] West CR, Harding JE, Williams CE, et al. Quantitative electroencephalographic patterns in normal preterm infants over the first week after birth. Early Hum Dev 2006;82(1):43–51.

[9] Klebermass K, Kuhle S, Olischar M, et al. Intra- and extrauterine maturation of amplitude-integrated electroencephalographic activity in preterm infants younger than 30 weeks of gestation. Biol Neonate 2006;89(2):120–5.

[10] Greisen G, Hellstrom-Westas L, Lou H, et al. EEG depression and germinal layer haemorrhage in the newborn. Acta Paediatr Scand 1987;76(3):519–25.

[11] Hellström-Westas L, Rosen I, Svenningsen NW. Cerebral function monitoring during the first week of life in extremely small low birthweight (ESLBW) infants. Neuropediatrics 1991;22(1):27–32.

[12] Inder TE, Buckland L, Williams CE, et al. Lowered electroencephalographic spectral edge frequency predicts the presence of cerebral white matter injury in premature infants. Pediatrics 2003;111(1):27–33.

[13] Barker DP, Rutter N. Exposure to invasive procedures in neonatal intensive care unit admissions. Arch Dis Child Fetal Neonatal Ed 1995;72(1):F47–8.

[14] Als H, Duffy FH, McAnulty GB, et al. Early experience alters brain function and structure. Pediatrics 2004;113(4):846–57.

[15] Lombroso CT. Neonatal polygraphy in full-term and premature infants: a review of normal and abnormal findings. J Clin Neurophysiol 1985;2(2):105–55.

[16] Connell JA, Oozeer R, Dubowitz V. Continuous 4-channel EEG monitoring: a guide to interpretation, with normal values, in preterm infants. Neuropediatrics 1987;18(3):138–45.

[17] Lamblin MD, Andre M, Challamel MJ, et al. Electroencephalography of the premature and term newborn. Maturational aspects and glossary. Neurophysiol Clin 1999;29(2):123–219.

[18] Selton D, Andre M, Hascoet JM. Normal EEG in very premature infants: reference criteria. Clin Neurophysiol 2000;111(12):2116–24.

[19] Hayakawa M, Okumura A, Hayakawa F, et al. Background electroencephalographic (EEG) activities of very preterm infants born at less than 27 weeks gestation: a study on the degree of continuity. Arch Dis Child Fetal Neonatal Ed 2001;84(3):F163–7.

[20] Vecchierini MF, d'Allest AM, Verpillat P. EEG patterns in 10 extreme premature neonates with normal neurological outcome: qualitative and quantitative data. Brain Dev 2003;25(5): 330–7.

[21] Victor S, Appleton RE, Beirne M, et al. Spectral analysis of electroencephalography in premature newborn infants: normal ranges. Pediatr Res 2005;57(3):336–41.

[22] Benda GI, Engel RC, Zhang YP. Prolonged inactive phases during the discontinuous pattern of prematurity in the electroencephalogram of very-low-birthweight infants. Electroencephalogr Clin Neurophysiol 1989;72(3):189–97.

[23] Viniker DA, Maynard DE, Scott DF. Cerebral function studies in neonates. Clin Electroencephalogr 1984;15(4):185–92.

[24] Verma UL, Archbald F, Tejani NA, et al. Cerebral function monitor in the neonate. I: normal patterns. Dev Med Child Neurol 1984;26(2):154–61.

[25] Thornberg E, Thiringer K. Normal pattern of the cerebral function monitor trace in term and preterm neonates. Acta Paediatr Scand 1990;79(1):20–5.

[26] Hellström-Westas L, Rosén I, de Vries LS, et al. Amplitude-integrated EEG: classification and interpretation in preterm and term infants. Neoreviews 2006;7:e76–87.

[27] Hellström-Westas L, Inghammar M, Isaksson K, et al. Short term effects of incubator covers on quiet sleep in stable preterm infants. Acta Paediatr 2001;90(9):1004–8.

[28] Westrup B, Hellström-Westas L, Stjernqvist K, et al. No indications of increased quiet sleep in infants who received care based on the Newborn Individualized Developmental Care and Assessment Program (NIDCAP). Acta Paediatr 2002;91(3):318–22.

[29] Greisen G, Hellström-Westas L, Lou H, et al. Sleep-waking shifts and cerebral blood flow in stable preterm infants. Pediatr Res 1985;19(11):1156–9.

[30] Scher MS, Johnson MW, Holditch-Davis D. Cyclicity of neonatal sleep behaviors at 25 to 30 weeks' postconceptional age. Pediatr Res 2005;57(6):879–82.

[31] Watanabe K, Hakamada S, Kuroyanagi M, et al. Electroencephalographical study of intraventricular hemorrhage in the preterm infant. Neuropediatrics 1983;14(4):225–30.

[32] Clancy RR, Tharp BR, Enzman D. EEG in premature infants with intraventricular hemorrhage. Neurology 1984;34(5):583–90.

[33] Connell J, Oozeer R, Regev R, et al. Continuous four-channel EEG monitoring in the evaluation of echodense ultrasound lesions and cystic leukomalacia. Arch Dis Child 1987;62(10): 1019–24.

[34] Connell J, deVries L, Oozeer R, et al. Predictive value of early continuous electroencephalogram monitoring in ventilated preterm infants with intraventricular hemorrhage. Pediatrics 1988;82(3):337–43.

[35] Aso K, Abdad-Barmada M, Scher MS. EEG and the neuropathology in premature neonates with intraventricular hemorrhage. J Clin Neurophysiol 1993;10(3):304–13.

[36] Watanabe K, Hayakawa F, Okumura A, Neonatal EEG. a powerful tool in the assessment of brain damage in preterm infants. Brain Dev 1999;21(6):361–72.

[37] Hayakawa F, Okumura A, Kato T, et al. Determination of timing of brain injury in preterm infants with periventricular leukomalacia with serial neonatal electroencephalography. Pediatrics 1999;104(5 Pt1):1077–81.

[38] Biagioni E, Bartalena L, Biver P, et al. Electroencephalographic dysmaturity in preterm infants: a prognostic tool in the early postnatal period. Neuropediatrics 1996;27(6):311–6.

[39] Marret S, Parain D, Jeannot E, et al. Positive rolandic sharp waves in the EEG of the premature newborn: a five year prospective study. Arch Dis Child 1992;67(7):948–51.

[40] Hellstrom-Westas L, Bell AH, Skov L, et al. Cerebroelectrical depression following surfactant treatment in preterm neonates. Pediatrics 1992;89(4 Pt1):643–7.

[41] Bell AH, Greisen G, Pryds O. Comparison of the effects of phenobarbitone and morphine administration on EEG activity in preterm babies. Acta Paediatr 1993;82(1):35–9.

[42] Young GB, da Silva OP. Effects of morphine on the electroencephalograms of neonates: a prospective, observational study. Clin Neurophysiol 2000;111(11):1955–60.

[43] Nguyen The Tich S, Vecchierini MF, Debillon T, et al. Effects of sufentanil on electroencephalogram in very and extremely preterm neonates. Pediatrics 2003;111(1):123–8.

[44] Greisen G, Pryds O. Low CBF, discontinuous EEG activity, and periventricular brain injury in ill, preterm neonates. Brain Dev 1989;11(3):164–8.

[45] Greisen G, Pryds O, Rosen I, et al. Poor reversibility of EEG abnormality in hypotensive, preterm neonates. Acta Paediatr Scand 1988;77:785–90.

[46] West CR, Groves AM, Williams CE, et al. Early low cardiac output is associated with compromised electroencephalographic activity in very preterm infants. Pediatr Res 2006; 59(4 Pt 1):610–5.

[47] Benders MJ, Meinesz JH, van Bel F, et al. Changes in electrocortical brain activity during exchange transfusions in newborn infants. Biol Neonate 2000;78(1):17–21.

[48] Kurtis PS, Rosenkrantz TS, Zalneraitis EL. Cerebral blood flow and EEG changes in preterm infants with patent ductus arteriosus. Pediatr Neurol 1995;12(2):114–9.

[49] Eaton DG, Wertheim D, Oozeer R, et al. Reversible changes in cerebral activity associated with acidosis in preterm neonates. Acta Paediatr 1994;83(5):486–92.

[50] Victor S, Appleton RE, Beirne M, et al. Effect of carbon dioxide on background cerebral electrical activity and fractional oxygen extraction in very low birth weight infants just after birth. Pediatr Res 2005;58(3):579–85.

[51] Hellström-Westas L, de Vries LS, Rosén I. An atlas on amplitude integrated EEGs in the newborn. London: Parthenon Publishing; 2003.

[52] Stenninger E, Eriksson E, Stigfur A, et al. Monitoring of early postnatal glucose homeostasis and cerebral function in newborn infants of diabetic mothers. A pilot study. Early Hum Dev 2001;62(1):23–32.

[53] Pryds O, Christensen NJ, Friis-Hansen B. Increased cerebral blood flow and plasma epinephrine in hypoglycemic, preterm neonates. Pediatrics 1990;85(2):172–6.

[54] Gluckman PD, Wyatt JS, Azzopardi D, et al. Selective head cooling with mild systemic hypothermia after neonatal encephalopathy: multicentre randomised trial. Lancet 2005; 365(9460):663–70.

[55] Tharp BR, Scher MS, Clancy RR. Serial EEGs in normal and abnormal infants with birthweights less than 1200 grams - a prospective study with long term follow-up. Neuropediatrics 1989;20(2):64–72.

[56] Hayakawa M, Okumura A, Hayakawa F, et al. Nutritional state and growth and functional maturation of the brain in extremely low birth weight infants. Pediatrics 2003;111(5 Pt 1): 991–5.

[57] Scher MS, Alvin J, Gaus L, et al. Uncoupling of EEG-clinical neonatal seizures after antiepileptic drug use. Pediatr Neurol 2003;28(4):277–80.

[58] Bye AM, Flanagan D. Spatial and temporal characteristics of neonatal seizures. Epilepsia 1995;36(10):1009–16.

ELSEVIER
SAUNDERS

CLINICS IN
PERINATOLOGY

Clin Perinatol 33 (2006) 649–665

Prolonged Electroencephalogram Monitoring for Seizures and Their Treatment

Robert R. Clancy, MD

University of Pennsylvania School of Medicine, The Children's Hospital of Philadelphia,
34th Street and Civic Center Boulevard, Philadelphia, PA 19104, USA

Background

Examining cerebral cortical function in an awake, cooperative adult is a reasonably easy, straightforward task. Cognitive function can be reliably determined by the assessment of orientation, receptive and expressive language, memory, problem solving, mathematical skills, and proverb interpretation. These traditional cognitive tasks are sensitive measures of the integrity of cerebral cortical functioning. In contrast, the same task is daunting in even the healthiest newborn infants. Even in an awake, well newborn infant, no reliable bedside clinical tools demonstrate the health of the cerebral cortex. Because the electroencephalogram (EEG) is exclusively generated by the outermost layers of the cerebral cortex, careful examination of the integrity of the EEG is a sensitive, albeit nonspecific yardstick for measuring the health of the cortex of the immature central nervous system [1]. In the past decades, many studies have confirmed the value of routine neonatal EEG examinations in assessing brain maturity, sleep cycling, the presence and severity of encephalopathy, and seizures [2–4].

Seizures, which arise from the cerebral cortex, are an important clinical sign in the neurology of the neonate [5]. The unique neurobiology of the immature brain, with its rather luxurious excitatory circuits compared with its sparse inhibitory circuits, renders the neonate uniquely vulnerable to seizures [6–8]. The neonatal period eclipses all other epochs of the human life span for the highest incidence of seizures [9–12]. Furthermore, studies have empirically established that infants who experience seizures face substantially higher mortality and morbidity rates than those who do not

E-mail address: Clancy@email.chop.edu

[13–17]. Thus, an intimate connection exists between EEG monitoring for neonatal seizures and the quest to evaluate the health of the cerebral cortex.

Diagnosing seizures in the human newborn can be exceedingly difficult, even for experienced observers. The outward manifestations of seizures may be subtle and overlooked, even on careful inspection. The drama of the full-blown generalized tonic clonic seizure is rarely witnessed in the neonatal intensive care unit (NICU). Some clinical seizure manifestations may incorporate movements, activities, or behaviors that mimic the natural repertoire of the healthy infant. Examples include innocent startles, stretching, hiccups, or the behaviors of rapid-eye-movement sleep (called *active sleep* in neonates). In neonates requiring iatrogenic paralysis with neuromuscular blocking agents to optimize cardiorespiratory care, clinical seizures cannot be witnessed except for episodic autonomic changes, such as paroxysmal tachycardia or blood pressure spikes [18–20]. Even in nonparalyzed infants, only approximately 20% of electrographic neonatal seizures provoke clinical signs [14,21]. In some infants, all seizures are subclinical even in the absence of therapeutic paralysis. Consequently, without an EEG, accurately quantifying the presence, number, and duration of seizures in the newborn is extremely difficult.

Fig. 1 illustrates the incomplete overlap of EEG and clinical seizures in the neonate. Most electrographic seizures arise subclinically and do not provoke visible, distinctive clinical or autonomic changes. However, many abnormal, paroxysmal clinical attacks ("seizures" in the broadest, most generic use of the term) manifested by some sick neonates are not specifically provoked by coincidental electrographic seizures. Examples include nonepileptic opisthotonic posturing or motor stereotypies such as "bicycling

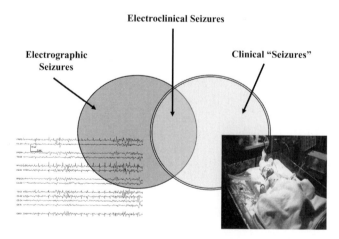

Fig. 1. An incomplete overlap between electrographic and clinical seizures occurs in neonates. Most electrographic neonatal seizures do not provoke distinctive attacks of clinical seizures. Some clinical "seizures" are not epileptic and do not show coincident ictal EEG activity. *Electroclinical seizures* refer to clinical seizures specifically triggered by electrographic seizures.

movements" of the legs [22–24]. Some experts believe that these paroxysmal clinical attacks represent primitive brainstem motor subroutines that are pathologically released during serious brain disease. Although these clinical events are clearly abnormal and arise in critically ill children, they are not epileptic in character and are unlikely to respond to treatment with antiepileptic drugs (AEDs). Finally, electroclinical seizures also occur in which distinctive abnormal clinical signs, such as repetitive clonic jerking of the face or arm musculature, correlate uniquely with simultaneous electrographic seizures demonstrated on the EEG. Because of the difficulties with clinical recognition of neonatal seizures, the EEG is generally regarded as the gold standard for confirming the presence of epileptic seizures and quantifying their burden. In addition, the interictal EEG background provides important information that describes the health of the neonatal cortex between seizures [25].

Routine electroencephalogram examinations

Routine EEG examinations can be performed in the EEG laboratory or at the patient's bedside, even in the electronically hostile environment of the intensive care unit (ICU). Routine EEG examinations are initiated and personally overseen by a recording technologist and typically last approximately 30 minutes. The advantages of routine EEG examinations are that they are directly supervised by a knowledgeable, certified technologist and interpreted by a qualified electroencephalographer. This brief study provides a highly detailed, albeit brief, picture of the ongoing EEG background. The EEG background is a "stage," the moment-to-moment cerebral electrical activity, against which transient EEG patterns (eg, sharp waves) or transient sustained events (eg, electrographic seizures) arise. Even these brief 30-minute snapshots of the EEG background are prognostically helpful [2–4]. Markedly abnormal backgrounds, such as isoelectric (flat) or burst-suppression tracings, are highly predictive of adverse outcomes, including death and chronic static encephalopathy. Fig. 2 shows the markedly abnormal pattern of burst suppression, in which the background invariantly alternates between brief bursts of abnormal electric signals and longer periods of low voltage suppression. Distinctive brief EEG transients, such as potentially epileptogenic discharges (Fig. 3) that may indicate a lowered seizure threshold [26] and positive rolandic or vertex sharp waves [27,28] that may indicate periventricular leukomalacia, can be seen easily on routine EEG recordings. These brief electrical transients are unlikely to be seen in EEG formats that temporally compress the EEG display. Furthermore, the presence of marked EEG background activity implies substantial EEG dysfunction, predicting future electrographic seizures. This finding was shown by Laroia and colleagues [29] in a prospective study in which they performed prolonged EEG monitoring in predetermined high-risk neonatal populations, such as

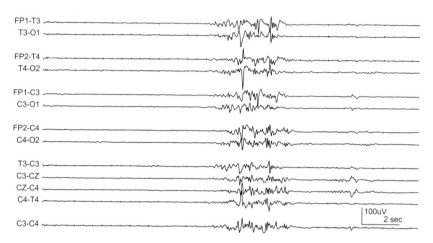

Fig. 2. Rhythm strip showing a markedly abnormal type of EEG background termed *burst suppression*, in which high-amplitude bursts of abnormal-appearing electrical activity invariantly alternate with low-voltage suppression. This pattern is not ictal and is not etiologically specific. It can be seen in a wide variety of severe, diffuse, acute brain disorders, such as hypoxic ischemic encephalopathy, severe trauma, and neonatal meningitis.

those with hypoxic ischemic encephalopathy. In infants whose early EEG background was significantly abnormal, 22 of 27 (81%) subsequently displayed electrographic seizures. In contrast, only 1 of 24 (4%) infants whose early background was normal or only immature showed subsequent seizures. These differences were highly significant.

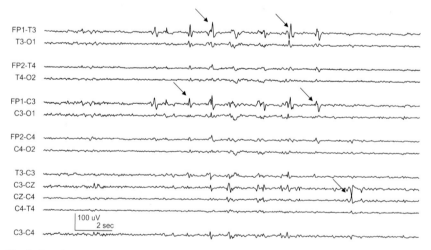

Fig. 3. Routine EEG examinations can provide important clues, such as potentially epileptogenic discharges (*arrows*) identified by their sharp morphology, excessive number, and tendency to recur in brief runs or trains. These discharges imply instability of the EEG and a tendency to develop actual electrographic seizures. They are likely to be missed in EEG display formats that temporally compress the EEG.

Nevertheless, conventional EEG examinations have important disadvantages. The test is ideally performed by a trained technologist who must carefully position the electrodes according to the international 10-20 system, modified for neonates (Fig. 4). Likewise, proper interpretation requires the availability of a specially trained electroencephalographer who is familiar with the nuances of neonatal EEG. Routine tracings may be very difficult, if not impossible, to obtain at night and during the weekends. Furthermore, their short duration implies that episodic events such as seizures may be missed unless a high frequency of seizures occurs.

The concept of prolonged EEG monitoring of the neonate is not new [30,31]. However, the task was extremely laborious in the past. With the development of high-speed digital technology, long-term video-EEG recordings have become more widely available at some medical centers. However, they are not considered customary care and many studies are confined to research applications. The advantage of digital video-EEG technology is that it combines a simultaneous video image of the patient with time-synchronized coincident EEG. These studies can be continued for days and stored to external hard drives or exported to central computer servers for review within or outside the hospital. They can be reviewed in real time and large data sets can be efficiently studied. For example, an uncomplicated 24-hour video-EEG examination can be reviewed within an hour. If necessary, it is even possible for the electroencephalographer to review studies at remote sites through the Internet. However, this connection is much slower and requires much logistical collaboration among the hospital's information systems, ICU personnel, the EEG laboratory, and the electroencephalographer. The disadvantages are that it still requires skilled

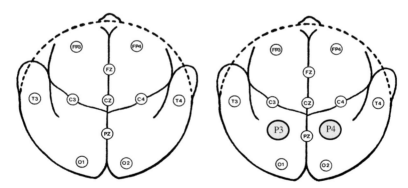

Fig. 4. The international 10-20 system, modified for neonates, provides guidelines for a reproducible and accurate distribution of scalp electrodes in routine EEG examination. All major brain locations are sampled, including the midline vertices and left and right frontal polar, central, temporal, and occipital regions (*left*). In contrast, the simplest amplitude integrated EEG study typically records from a single electrode pair in the left and right parietal areas (P3 and P4) (*right*).

EEG technologists and EEG readers to perform and review the study, it is expensive to implement and time-consuming to review, and most hospitals do not provide instant access to the technology. Thus, like routine EEG, a substantial delay may occur between the time the monitoring is first needed and when it is actually applied to the patient.

Long-term monitoring for electrographic seizures

One of the most common goals of long-term video-EEG monitoring is to detect the presence and burden of electrographic seizures. This approach has the same intention as long-term EEG monitoring in adult ICUs, where monitoring reveals the presence of electrographic seizures in a significant percentage of comatose or critically ill patients [32,33]. The criteria used to identify electrographic seizures in neonates have important differences, however, compared with those used for older children or adults. An electrographic neonatal seizure (ENS) is defined as a distinct electrographic event with a definite beginning, middle, and end [34]. The minimum seizure duration is conventionally cited as 10 seconds and the minimum amplitude that defines the beginning and end of the seizure is 2 μV. Typically, ENSs begin focally and evolve in amplitude and waveform morphology. They commonly migrate from their place of origin to adjacent areas and even to remote regions of the opposite hemisphere. ENSs have no single morphology and their appearance varies among individuals (Fig. 5). Their behavior as sustained, evolving electrographic events reveal their epileptic identity. Although electrographic seizures can occur in the context of a normal, moderately abnormal, or markedly abnormal EEG background, they are most likely to occur in the context of severely abnormal studies [25,29].

Currently, no consensus exists as to how to best quantify the burden of ENSs. A simple dichotomous diagnosis indicates only that seizures are either present or absent. However, this method gives no measure of their number, duration, or spatial distribution. The next level of quantification would be seizure counts, in which the number of ENSs is simply reported and frequency calculated (eg, five ENSs per hour). However, because electrographic seizures differ in their duration, this method does not provide a fully accurate picture of the seizure burden. Although the minimum duration of an electrographic seizure is 10 seconds, most last longer. The next level of complexity for quantifying neonatal seizure burden would include not only a seizure count but also the duration of each seizure. From these data, one could calculate the percentage of time that the focal ENS appeared in at least one brain location. Finally, a temporal–spatial analysis of electrographic seizures could be performed, measuring the duration of each electrographic seizure at each spatial location in the brain. This technique is extremely time-consuming and tedious, but provides a comprehensive representation of the number, duration, and spatial extent of the ENSs [35].

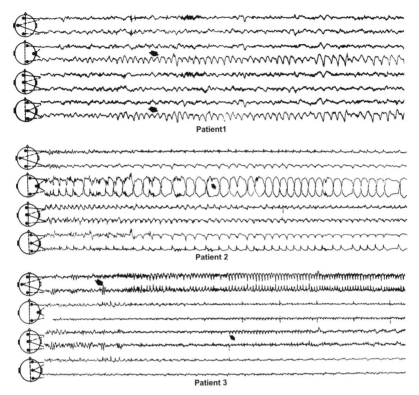

Fig. 5. Electrographic neonatal seizures vary in their appearance among these three neonatal patients (*arrows*). No single appearance identifies electrographic seizures. Rather, they are recognized by their behavior as stereotyped, evolving electrographic events that have a clear beginning, middle, and end.

The Children's Hospital of Philadelphia study of prolonged electroencephalogram monitoring after newborn heart surgery

Experts have long recognized that neonatal seizures occur in certain high-risk populations, such as those who had birth trauma, hypoxic ischemic encephalopathy, intracranial infections, or surgery for congenital heart defects (CHD) [36]. Although the incidence of seizures after newborn heart surgery has progressively declined (Table 1), a substantial number of patients still develop seizures in the immediate postoperative period. In some studies of survivors after surgery for CHD, postoperative seizures were a marker for poorer performance on follow-up neurodevelopmental tests [37–39].

A study was recently completed at The Children's Hospital of Philadelphia to define the contemporary incidence of postoperative seizures in a large group of children undergoing newborn heart surgery for serious forms of CHDs [40,41]. These children were participating in a larger study examining

Table 1
Historical overview of seizure incidence after newborn heart surgery

Series	Era	Subjects (N)	Clinical seizures	EEG seizures	Comments
Scattered report [63,64]	before 1985		<50%		
CHOP HLHS autopsy series [65]	1980–1985	50	32%		
Boston circulatory arrest trial [37]	1988–1992	170	6.4% (11/170)	19.8% (27/136)	TGA only
Boston alpha-vs. pH-stat [66]	1992–1996	182	4.5% (7/153)	7.1% (11/153)	TGA, TOF & VSD
CHOP allopurinol trial [67]	1992–1997	350	22% (15/67) 18% (33/187)	→ →	HLHS Placebo Non-HLHS (placebo & allopurinol)
CHOP apo-E polymorphisms study [41]	2001–2003	183	none	11.5% (21/183)	Mixed forms of CHDs

Abbreviations: CHOP, Children's Hospital of Philadelphia; HLHS, hypoplastic left heart syndrome; TGA, transposition of the great arteries; TOF, tetralogy of Fallot; VSD, ventricular septal defect.

the relationship between polymorphisms of the apolipoprotein E gene and subsequent neurodevelopmental outcome [42]. During the period of that study (2001–2003), 183 infants were examined postoperatively for 48 hours through video EEG. So that no potential patient subjects were missed, three portable research video EEG machines were acquired and used. Scalp surface electrodes were attached using collodion glue preoperatively and a brief 15-minute EEG baseline was obtained. Tracings were not obtained intraoperatively while the patient was on cardiopulmonary bypass (CPB) or during hypothermic circulatory arrest (HTCA). The studies were resumed after the children returned to the cardiac ICU from the operating room. As expected, the immediate postoperative EEG initially showed clear background abnormalities reflecting the medical status of the infants: they had just undergone the major stresses of cardiac surgery, CPB, HTCA, general anesthesia, and hypothermia (Fig. 6). The studies were continued for a minimum duration of 48 hours postoperatively and were reviewed for seizures every 12 hours. If ENSs were present, they were reported to the attending physician who decided the choice and dose of an AED, usually phenobarbital. Video-EEG monitoring was extended beyond the 48 hours of the research period to assist in the clinical management of some patients who experienced refractory seizures. MRI examinations were performed 7 to 10 days after surgery in most patients who exhibited postoperative ENSs, and the results correlated with video-EEG data, particularly regarding the site of origin of the seizures.

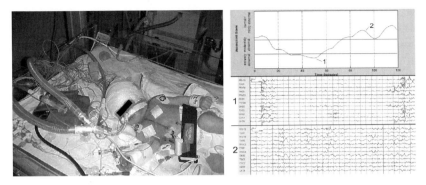

Fig. 6. In The Children's Hospital of Philadelphia video-EEG monitoring study, neonates were monitored for 48 hours after newborn heart surgery. The EEG background varied considerably in the postoperative period, reflecting their unsettled medical and physiologic states. The trends in EEG background changes are displayed by an investigation neonatal EEG monitoring device (*Courtesy of* Moberg Research, Inc., Ambler, Pennsylvania).

Of the 183 patients, 11.5% showed one or more electrographic seizures [41]. The onset of the first seizure ranged from 10 to 36 hours postoperatively (mean time of onset, 21 ± 6 hours). The total number of ENSs recorded during the 48-hour monitoring period ranged from 1 to 217 (mean, 72 ± 76 seizures). The maximum number of ENSs per hour ranged from 1 to 16 (mean, 7 ± 5 ENSs per hour). Post-hoc analysis of the sites of origin of the ENS was conducted by a simplified electrode array in which the complete EEG was reduced to five nonoverlapping regions of interest (Fig. 7). The site of origin of each seizure was determined using these five

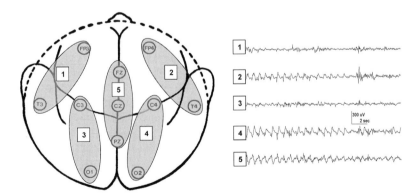

Fig. 7. This reduced array of electrode pairs is a subset of the full neonatal 10-20 system. Five nonoverlapping regions of interest sample the midline and both hemispheres symmetrically. This array simplifies identification of the sites of origin of electrographic seizures. The EEG sample shows electrographic seizure activity in regions 2, 4, and 5.

regions of interest. Most seizures appeared to arise from a single region of interest, but some appeared to arise simultaneously in more than one region. The sites of origin of the electrographic seizures were compared with the patterns of injury detected by the postoperative MRI scans. Reasonable correlations were seen between findings on the MRI examinations and the sites of origin of the ENSs. For example, children who showed diffuse acute injury (such as multifocal periventricular leukomalacia) had multiple sites from which individual seizures could arise. On the other hand, in children who had an exquisitely localized injury (such as a restricted infarct), all seizures arose from a single corresponding location.

Medical treatment of neonatal seizures

An old clinical adage states, "Treat the patient, not the EEG." Although this maxim may still be applicable to some clinical situations, it is outdated in the treatment of neonatal seizures. The goal of AED treatment in this context is to completely eliminate electrographic seizures. Because clinical recognition and quantification of seizures are notoriously difficult and unreliable, the real goal of drug treatment is the total elimination of ENSs determined by EEG monitoring. Thus, the EEG serves as the gold standard not only to establish the presence of seizures and quantify them but also to demonstrate the efficacy of treatment.

Phenobarbital is the traditional choice of neurologists and neonatologists worldwide for treating neonatal seizures. Unfortunately, this widespread clinical practice is not founded on a firm scientific basis. No formal, prospective, randomized, placebo-controlled trial has ever shown the efficacy of phenobarbital in treating acute neonatal seizures, and the medical literature fails to provide clear support for its use. Goldberg and colleagues [43] reported a randomized controlled study of thiopental administered soon after perinatal asphyxia. EEG examinations were not routinely performed and neonatal seizures were diagnosed on clinical grounds. Seizures were diagnosed in 76% of treated infants and 73% of placebo-treated controls. However, this study really examined the prevention of incipient seizures rather than the treatment of established seizures. More recently, Hall and colleagues [44] reported the results of a neuroprotection trial in which high-dose phenobarbital was administered to neonates who experienced perinatal asphyxia. The group receiving phenobarbital showed an insignificantly lower occurrence of seizures than the placebo group. Nevertheless, the phenobarbital group performed better on subsequent neurodevelopmental follow-up.

Connell and colleagues [45] reported the response to AEDs of ENSs detected during continuous EEG monitoring in 31 acutely ill neonates. Only 2 infants showed a complete cessation of both clinical and EEG seizures, and 6 others showed an equivocal electroclinical response. Clinical cessation of seizures occurred in 13 infants, although their electrographic seizures persisted. Weiner and colleagues [46] and others have reported this phenomenon of *uncoupling*, in which AED administration suppresses clinical seizures despite the continuation of EEG seizures. Both clinical and EEG seizures persisted in the remaining 10 infants in Connell's study. Bye and Flanagan [47] also reported an equivocal response of electroclinical seizures to phenobarbital treatment. In an uncontrolled efficacy study of phenobarbital in the treatment of ENSs, Boylan and colleagues [48] administered a standard dose (40 mg/kg) to patients and then performed video-EEG monitoring. However, there was no control group. Eleven of 22 patients (50%) showed a cessation of seizures, and those who showed no response were randomized to treatment with either lignocaine or benzodiazepines as a second-line drug. Painter and colleagues [49] reported a comparative study of ENS responses in neonates randomized to treatment with either phenobarbital or phenytoin. Cessation of ENSs occurred in 43% of patients treated with phenobarbital and 45% of those treated with phenytoin. However, because a placebo-control arm was not part of the study, absolute efficacy could not be determined. In a similar trial, Conde and colleagues [50] reported an uncontrolled study in which ENSs persisted in 17 of 32 (53%) neonates treated with phenobarbital or phenytoin. However, seizures were reported to rapidly cease in all 13 infants who showed no response after administration of midazolam.

In their Cochrane review of the treatment of seizures in the neonate, Evans and Levene [51] state, "at the present time, anti-convulsant therapy administered in the immediate period following perinatal asphyxia cannot be recommended for routine clinical practice, other than in the treatment of prolonged or frequent clinical seizures." Most recently, Sankar and Painter [52] recently published an insightful editorial on the widespread but scientifically unsubstantiated clinical preference for phenobarbital in treating neonatal seizures ("after all these years, we still love what doesn't work") and declared a pressing need for rigorous clinical trials in this area of neonatal neurology.

In addition to those about efficacy, concerns are increasing about the safety of phenobarbital and other central nervous system depressant drugs used in the newborn infant. In immature animal models, exposure to alcohol, general anesthetic agents, and antiepileptic drugs such as phenobarbital have measurable adverse impacts on brain growth and development. The extent to which these findings apply to the very young human nervous system is unknown. Apoptotic neuronal death is a necessary physiologic process in the natural sequence of normal brain development and occurs most robustly during periods of rapid brain growth and luxurious synaptogenesis. Apoptosis is a desired phenomenon that sculpts brain formation and its interconnections. Experts are concerned, however, that suppression of synaptic neurotransmission through blockade of glutamate N-methyl d-aspartate (NMDA) receptors or activation of γ-aminobutyric acid type A (GABA$_A$) receptors may trigger excessive apoptotic neurodegeneration.

Jevtovic-Todorovic and colleagues [53] examined the effects of commonly used general anesthetic agents in doses required to achieve a surgical plane of anesthesia for 6 hours, using a combination of nitrous oxide, midazolam, and isofluorane in 7-day-old rats. Anesthetized animals experienced widespread apoptotic neurodegeneration, deficits in synaptic functioning, and persistent impairments in learning and memory. In a similar investigation, Bittigau and colleagues [54] showed that early exposure of the immature rodent brain to phenytoin, phenobarbital, diazepam, clonazepam, vigabatrin, and valproate (at levels that overlap with values used for seizure control in children) caused apoptotic neurodegeneration. Ohmori and colleagues [55] showed phenytoin neurotoxicity (induced cell death and faulty migration) on the granule and Purkinje cells in the developing mouse cerebellum. Olney and colleagues [56] speculated that the GABA-mimetic and NMDA antagonistic effects of ethanol are responsible for the cardinal clinical features of fetal alcohol syndrome (small brain and cognitive-behavioral abnormalities).

Not all AEDs have these effects in the immature central nervous system. Glier and colleagues [57] compared topiramate with phenobarbital, phenytoin, and valproate and found that at therapeutic doses, topiramate did not induce apoptotic neurodegeneration. At supratherapeutic doses (more than 50 mg/kg per dose), modest but significant neurotoxicity was observed, but not at levels encountered in clinical practice. If phenobarbital can be proven to be truly effective in terminating neonatal seizures, its future use might be justified despite the theoretical concern for accelerated programmed cell death. However, if phenobarbital is not found efficacious, then this common practice may be avoided in the future.

The newborn drug development initiative

Many scenarios exist for treating newborn infants wherein medications are selected from traditional practice and conventional wisdom that are not supported by prospective, randomized, placebo-controlled trials. The National Institute of Child Health and Human Development and the Food and Drug Administration recently collaborated to create the Newborn Drug Development Initiative (NDDI) to close the gaps in knowledge of pharmacologic treatment of neonates for pain management and cardiologic, respiratory, gastrointestinal, and neurologic disorders, including neonatal seizures. According to the recently published workshops sponsored by the NDDI, the Neurology Committee made recommendations suggesting the framework for future randomized controlled clinical trials to show the efficacy of phenobarbital for treating neonatal seizures [58].

Alternative forms of electroencephalogram monitoring

Cerebral function monitors are a class of EEG devices that have been simplified for use by bedside caregivers, including nurses and neonatologists.

This technology is not intended to replace traditional EEG, but rather to serve as a readily available bedside supplement that could be applied by non-neurologists with modest training. It provides valuable long-term tracking of cerebral function by a simplified single channel of EEG activity. One common method of monitoring is called *amplitude-integrated EEG* (aEEG), in which a single-channel EEG (eg, the left parietal to the right parietal region) can be displayed as a compressed signal showing valuable trends over time (Fig. 8) [59–61]. The main advantages of aEEG are that it is inexpensive and those directly caring for the patient can apply it quickly when

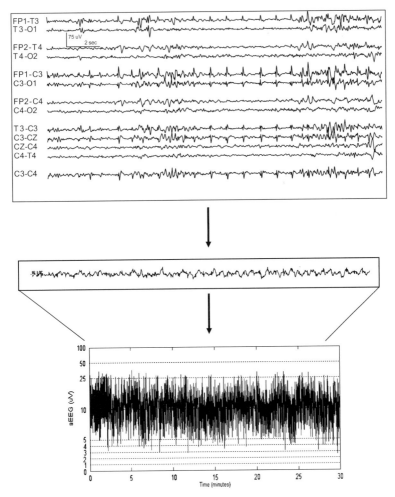

Fig. 8. The routine neonatal EEG examination typically displays 12 or more channels from the full array of the 10-20 system. Cerebral function monitors, such as aEEG, use a single channel from a pair of scalp electrodes (commonly the left and right parietal regions) and then processes the raw EEG to a compressed display, which is very useful for reviewing long-term trends.

necessary, without having to wait for EEG laboratory personnel to arrive at the bedside. aEEG compresses the time axis of the examination, displaying long-term trends that can easily be followed and conveniently reviewed. Some seizures can be recognized by distinctive elevation of the upper and lower margins of the recording.

aEEG also has some disadvantages. The shortage of formal training guidelines for use and interpretation of this technology may cause inexperienced users to "over-read" or "under-read" the studies [62]. Details of the EEG background will be missed, especially short-lived transient events such as sharp EEG transients, positive rolandic sharp waves, and focal slowing. Seizures that are brief, low amplitude, or spatially confined to the frontal-polar, temporal or occipital regions will not be visible on the one-channel aEEG. Single-channel aEEG recordings may also miss hemispheric asymmetries. Still, aEEG offers tremendous advantages and should be considered a valuable supplement to, rather than a replacement of, traditional EEG technology.

The future

An impressive evolution has occurred of biomedical technology to assess and track the status of the newborn brain. It should not be too difficult to blend the best features of traditional full-array video EEG with the simplicity and ease of use of cerebral function monitors such as aEEG. Technology is conceivable that will allow neonates to be recorded with nearly a full complement of electrodes, with the bedside examiner required to review only the simple one-channel aEEG. Later, electroencephalographers can review the study displayed in its traditional format. Computer-based neonatal seizure detection algorithms can be applied to the whole array of utilized electrodes to assist seizure detection, rather than having experts rely on visual inspection of a single aEEG signal alone. Furthermore, combining such flexible EEG technology with other relevant data, such as near-infrared spectroscopy and physiologic parameters (eg, mean arterial blood pressure, P_{CO_2}, and P_{O_2}), can provide a powerful alliance to assist the bedside clinician in optimizing the management of critically ill neonates. Much work remains to determine the full value of cerebral function monitoring. Hopefully, relevant clinical trials of the efficacy and safety of the AED treatment of neonatal seizures will soon be completed.

References

[1] Clancy R, Bergqvist AC, Dlugos D. Neonatal electroencephalography. In: Ebersole JS, Pedley T, editors. Current practice of clinical electroencephalography. Philadelphia: Lippincott Williams & Wilkins; 2003. p. 160–234.

[2] Holmes GL, Lombroso CT. Prognostic value of background patterns in the neonatal EEG. J Clin Neurophysiol 1993;10(3):323–52.

[3] Monod N, Pajot N, Guidasci S, The neonatal EEG. statistical studies and prognostic value in full-term and pre-term babies. Electroencephalogr Clin Neurophysiol 1972;32:529–44.

[4] Watanabe K, Hayakawa F, Okumura A. Neonatal EEG: a powerful tool in the assessment of brain damage in preterm infants. Brain Dev 1999;21(6):361–72.

[5] Volpe J. Neonatal seizures: current concepts and revised classification. Pediatrics 1989;84: 422–8.

[6] Jensen FE, Holmes GL, Lombroso CT, et al. Age-dependent changes in long-term seizure susceptibility and behavior after hypoxia in rats. Epilepsia 1992;33(6):971–80.

[7] Jensen FE, Blume H, Alvarado S, et al. NBQX blocks acute and late epileptogenic effects of perinatal hypoxia. Epilepsia 1995;36:966–72.

[8] Jensen FE. Acute and chronic effects of seizures in the developing brain: experimental models. Epilepsia 1999;40:S51–8.

[9] Eriksson M, Zetterstrom R. Neonatal convulsions. Incidence and causes in the Stockholm area. Acta Paediatra Scand 1979;68:807–11.

[10] Bergman I, Painter MJ, Hirsch RP. Outcomes in neonates with convulsions treated in an intensive care unit. Ann Neurol 1983;14:642.

[11] Lanska MJ, Lanska DJ, Baumann RJ, et al. A population-based study of neonatal seizures in Fayette County, Kentucky. Neurology 1995;45(4):724–32.

[12] Ronen GM, Penney S, Andrews W. The epidemiology of clinical neonatal seizures in Newfoundland: a population-based study. J Pediatr 1999;134(1):71–5.

[13] Legido A, Clancy RR, Berman PH. Neurologic outcome after electroencephalographically proven neonatal seizures. Pediatrics 1991;88(3):583–96.

[14] Mizrahi EM, Clancy R, Dunn JK, et al. Neurologic impairment, developmental delay and post-natal seizures two years after video-EEG documented seizures in near-term and full-term neonates: Report of the Clinical Research Centers for Neonatal Seizures. Epilepsia 2001;102:47.

[15] Ortibus EL, Sum JM, Hahn JS. Predictive value of EEG for outcome and epilepsy following neonatal seizures. Electroencephalogr Clin Neurophysiol 1996;98(3):175–85.

[16] Ellenberg J, Nelson K. Cluster of perinatal events identifying infants at high risk for death or disability. J Pediatr 1988;113:546–52.

[17] Nelson KB, Broman SH. Perinatal risk factors in children with serious motor and mental handicaps. Ann Neurol 1977;2(5):371–7.

[18] Perlman JM, Volpe JJ. Seizures in the preterm infant: effects on cerebral blood flow velocity, intracranial pressure, and arterial blood pressure. J Pediatr 1983;102(2):288–93.

[19] Goldberg R, Goldman S, Ramsay R. Detection of seizure activity in the paralyzed neonate using continuous monitoring. Pediatrics 1982;69:583–6.

[20] Lou H, Friss-Hansen B. Arterial blood pressure elevations during motor activity and epileptic seizures in the newborn. Acta Paediatra Scand 1979;68:803–6.

[21] Clancy R, Legido A, Lewis D. Occult neonatal seizures. Epilepsia 1988;29:256–61.

[22] Mizrahi EM, Kellaway P. Characterization and classification of neonatal seizures. Neurology 1987;37(12):1837–44.

[23] Mizrahi EM. Neonatal seizures: problems in diagnosis and classification. Epilepsia 1987; 28(Suppl 1):S46–55.

[24] Mizrahi EM, Kellaway P. Diagnosis and management of neonatal seizures. Philadelphia: Lippincott-Raven; 1998.

[25] Clancy R, Legido A. Neurologic outcome after EEG-proven neonatal seizures. Pediatr Res 1987;21:489A.

[26] Clancy R. Interictal sharp EEG transients in neonatal seizures. J Child Neurol 1989;4: 30–8.

[27] Marret S, Parain D, Jeannot E, et al. Positive rolandic sharp waves in the EEG of the premature newborn: a five year prospective study. Arch Dis Child 1992;67(7):948–51.

[28] Clancy R, Tharp BR. Positive rolandic sharp waves in the electroencephalograms of premature infants with intraventricular hemorrhage. Electroencephalogr Clin Neurophysiol 1984; 57:395–404.
[29] Laroia N, Guillet R, Burchfiel J, et al. EEG background as predictor of electrographic seizures in high-risk neonates. Epilepsia 1998;39(5):545–51.
[30] Tharp BR. Intensive video/EEG monitoring of neonates. Adv Neurol 1986;46:107–25.
[31] Coen RW, McCutchen C, Wermer D, et al. Continuous monitoring of the electroencephalogram following perinatal asphyxia. J Pediatr 1982;100:628–30.
[32] Claassen J, Mayer S, Kowalski G, et al. Detection of electrographic seizures with continuous EEG monitoring in critically ill patients. Neurology 2004;62:1743–8.
[33] Scheuer M. Continuous EEG monitoring in the intensive care unit. Epilepsia 2002;43(Suppl 1): 114–27.
[34] Clancy RR, Legido A. The exact ictal and interictal duration of electroencephalographic neonatal seizures. Epilepsia 1987;28(5):537–41.
[35] Clancy R, Mizrahi E. Neonatal seizures. In: Wyllie E, editor. The treatment of epilepsy. Philadelphia: Lippincott Williams & Wilkins; 2006. p. 487–510.
[36] Clancy RR, McGaurn S, Wernovsky G, et al. Risk of seizures in survivors of newborn heart surgery using deep hypothermic circulatory arrest. Pediatrics 2001;111:592–601.
[37] Newburger JW, Jonas JA, Wernovsky G. A comparison of the perioperative neurologic effects of hypothermic circulatory arrest versus low-flow cardiopulmonary bypass in infant heart surgery. N Engl J Med 1993;329:1057–64.
[38] Bellinger DC, Jonas RA, Rappaport LA, et al. Developmental and neurologic status of children after heart surgery with hypothermic circulatory arrest or low-flow cardiopulmonary bypass. N Engl J Med 1995;332(9):549–55.
[39] Bellinger DC, Wypij D, Kuban KCK, et al. Developmental and neurologic status of children at four years of age after heart surgery with hypothermic circulatory arrest or low-flow cardiopulmonary bypass. Circulation 1999;100:526–32.
[40] Gaynor JW, Nicolson SC, Jarvic G, et al. Increasing duration of deep hypothermic circulatory arrest is associated with an increased incidence of postoperative seizures. J Thorac Cardiovasc Surg 2005;130:1278–86.
[41] Clancy RR, Sharif U, Ichord R, et al. Electrographic neonatal seizures after infant heart surgery. Epilepsia 2005;46:84–90.
[42] Gaynor JW, Gerdes M, Zackai EH, et al. Apolipoprotein E genotype and neurodevelopmental sequelae of infant cardiac surgery. J Thorac Cardiovasc Surg 2003;126:1736–45.
[43] Goldberg RN, Moscoso P, Bauer CR, et al. Use of barbiturate therapy in severe perinatal asphyxia: A randomized controlled trial. J Pediatr 1986;109:851–6.
[44] Hall RT, Hall FK, Daily DK. High-dose phenobarbital therapy in term newborn infants with severe perinatal asphyxia: a randomized, prospective study with three-year follow-up. J Pediatr 1998;132(2):345–8.
[45] Connell J, Oozeer R, de Vries L, et al. Clinical and EEG response to anticonvulsants in neonatal seizures. Arch Dis Child 1989;64(4):459–64.
[46] Weiner SP, Painter MJ, Geva D, et al. Neonatal seizures: electroclinical dissociation. Pediatr Neurol 1991;7(5):363–8.
[47] Bye AM, Flanagan D. Spatial and temporal characteristics of neonatal seizures. Epilepsia 1995;36(10):1009–16.
[48] Boylan GB, Rennie JM, Pressler RM, et al. Phenobarbitone, neonatal seizures, and video-EEG. Arch Dis Child Fetal Neonatal Ed 2002;86(3):F165–70.
[49] Painter MJ, Scher MS, Stein AD, et al. Phenobarbital compared with phenytoin for the treatment of neonatal seizures. N Engl J Med 1999;341(7):485–9.
[50] Conde J, Borges A, Martinez E, et al. Midazolam in neonatal seizures with no response to phenobarbital. Neurology 2005;64:876–9.
[51] Evans DJ, Levene MI. Anticonvulsants for preventing mortality and morbidity in full term newborns with perinatal asphyxia. Cochrane Database Syst Rev 2001;3: CD001240.

[52] Sankar R, Painter M. Neonatal seizures: after all these years we still love what doesn't work. Neurology 2005;64:776–7.

[53] Jevtovic-Todorovic V, Hartman D, Izumi Y, et al. Early exposure to common anesthetic agents cause widespread neurodegeneration in the developing rat brain and persistent learning deficits. J Neurosci 2003;23:876–82.

[54] Bittigau P, Sifringer M, Genz K, et al. Antiepileptic drugs and apoptotic neurodegeneration in the developing brain. Proc Natl Acad Sci USA 2002;99:15089–94.

[55] Ohmori H, Ogura H, Yasuda M, et al. Developmental neurotoxicity of phenytoin on granule cells and Purkinje cells in mouse cerebellum. J Neurochem 1999;72:1497–506.

[56] Olney JW, Wozniak DF, Farber N, et al. The enigma of fetal alcohol neurotoxicity. Ann Med 2002;34:109–19.

[57] Glier C, Dzietko M, Bittigau P, et al. Therapeutic doses of topiramate are not toxic to the developing rat brain. Exp Neurol 2004;187:403–9.

[58] Clancy RR. Summary proceedings from the neurology group on neonatal seizures. Pediatrics 2006;117:s23–7.

[59] Toet MC, Hellstrom-Westas L, Groenendaal F, et al. Amplitude integrated EEG 3 and 6 hours after birth in full term neonates with hypoxic-ischaemic encephalopathy. Arch Dis Child Fetal Neonatal Ed 1999;81(1):F19–23.

[60] de Vries L, Hellstrom-Westas L. Role of cerebral function monitoring in the newborn. Arch Dis Child Fetal Neonatal Ed 2005;90:F201–7.

[61] Hellstrom-Westas L, Klette H, Thorngren-Jerneck K, et al. Early prediction of outcome with a-EEG in preterm infants with large intraventricular hemorrhages. Neuropediatrics 2001; 32(6):319–24.

[62] Rennie J, Chorley G, Boylan G, et al. Non-expert use of the cerebral function monitor for neonatal seizure detection. Arch Dis Child Fetal Neonatal Ed 2004;89:F37.

[63] Ferry P. Neurologic sequelae of open-heart surgery in children: an irritating question. Am J Dis Child 1990;144:369–73.

[64] Ferry P. Neurologic sequelae of cardiac surgery in children. Am J Dis Child 1987;141: 309–12.

[65] Glauser TA, Rorke LB, Weinberg AD, et al. Acquired neuropathological lesions associated with the hypoplastic left heart syndrome. Pediatrics 1990;85:991–1000.

[66] Bellinger DC, Wypij D, du Plessis AJ, et al. Developmental and neurological effects of alpha-stat versus ph-stat strategies for deep hypothermic cardiopulmonary bypass in infants. J Thorac Cardiovasc Surg 2001;121:374–83.

[67] Clancy RR, McGaurn SA, Goin JE, et al. Allopurinol neuro-cardiac protection trial in infants undergoing heart surgery utilizing deep hypothermic circulatory arrest. Pediatrics 2001;107:61–70.

ELSEVIER
SAUNDERS

CLINICS IN
PERINATOLOGY

Clin Perinatol 33 (2006) 667–677

Training Neonatal Staff in Recording and Reporting Continuous Electroencephalography

Andrew Whitelaw, MD, FRCPCH[a],*,
Robert D. White, MD[b]

[a]Neonatal Medicine, University of Bristol Medical School, Southmead Hospital,
Bristol BS10 5NB, United Kingdom
[b]Regional Neonatal Program, Memorial Hospital, 615 North Michigan Street,
South Bend, IN 46601, USA

Electroencephalography is now a neonatal clinical tool

Neonatal mortality has reached such low levels in developed countries that the emphasis in neonatology is shifting toward protection of the brain from the many potential threats in the perinatal period. Appreciation of the vulnerability of the brain and the recognition in real-time of changes in brain function are part of the creation of a culture of "brain-oriented neonatal intensive care," a phrase that was proposed first by the pioneer Swedish neonatologist, Neils Svenningsen in 1982 [1]. As practicing neonatologists who have been using continuous electroencephalography (EEG) for some years in neonatal intensive care, the authors believe that sufficient data have now become available to confirm that this technique is practical, diagnostic, and prognostic in neonatal intensive care. For us, continuous EEG has grown from being purely a research tool for investigators to being a useful clinical tool that complements neurologic examination, neuroimaging, and biochemical analyses.

The need for training of neonatal staff in electroencephalography

The history of neonatology is replete with examples of promising new technology that transitions from research to clinical application in a manner that is regulated poorly and susceptible to overuse or misuse. Technology that is expensive, complex, and for which there is a limited application

---

* Corresponding author.
E-mail address: andrew.whitelaw@bristol.ac.uk (A. Whitelaw).

doi:10.1016/j.clp.2006.06.006

(eg, extracorporeal membrane oxygenation, heart transplantation) may be less likely to be used inappropriately, but less expensive and simple technologies for which many potential applications are apparent carry a considerable risk for misuse in their early stages (eg, ventilators, high-frequency oscillators, inhaled nitric oxide).

To be able to provide a competent service to record continuous EEG and to interpret the results 24 hours a day require that several neonatal staff are trained adequately and can report EEG findings in a structured, reproducible, and evidence-based manner. The authors propose that appropriate training would require the sequence described in Box 1.

Preliminary training

Before taking delivery of equipment, clinicians should establish a solid scientific background by reading *An Atlas of Amplitude-Integrated EEGs in the Newborn* [2]; reviewing recent papers, including this issue of the *Clinics*

Box 1. Suggested sequence to establish the "learning curve" for continuous electroencephalography monitor interpretation in the neonatal ICU

- Before taking delivery of EEG equipment, establish scientific background by:
  reading *An Atlas of Amplitude-Integrated EEGs in the Newborn* and this issue of the *Clinics in Perinatology*
  reviewing recent papers
  attending pertinent conferences
  contacting one or more experienced mentors
- Upon delivery of equipment, all clinicians should attend a comprehensive in-service by the manufacturer's representative.
- As soon as equipment is used clinically, daily "EEG review" sessions should be established so that all clinical staff quickly can become aware of common patterns, artifacts, and so forth.
- There should be ongoing review of challenging tracings/cases with mentors.
- Soon after beginning use of the equipment, at least one clinician from each institution should attend a formal training course.
- A system for regular review and discussion of new abstracts and articles should be established.
- At least annually, all clinicians who are involved in interpretation of continuous EEG recordings should participate in sessions that present multiple "unknown" tracings to check the accuracy of their interpretations.

in Perinatology and several of the key references for each article in this issue; attending pertinent conferences; and contacting one or more experienced mentors who will be available to help with the learning curve. Upon delivery of EEG equipment, all clinicians should attend a comprehensive in-service by the manufacturer's representative.

Early clinical use

An important element to establish as soon as continuous EEG monitoring is used clinically is the use of daily "EEG review" sessions so that all clinical staff quickly can become aware of common patterns, artifacts, and so forth with ongoing review of challenging tracings/cases with mentors. Soon after beginning, one or more clinicians also should attend a formal training course, such as that described below, and disseminate the information that is learned there to the clinical team back home.

Continuing education

The volume of abstracts and articles that describes the use of continuous EEG monitoring in newborns is growing rapidly, so a regular program for review and discussion of new findings should be established. At least annually, those clinicians who regularly interpret continuous EEG tracings also should participate in sessions that present multiple "unknown" tracings to check the accuracy of their interpretations.

We have recognized the need for training of neonatal medical staff and one of the authors (AW) has developed a 1-day course that is aimed at neonatal medical staff with knowledge of neonatology but limited personal hands-on experience of neonatal EEG.

One-day introductory interactive course in neonatal electroencephalography

The Bristol 1-day course "Cerebral Function Monitoring and Neurophysiology for Neonatologists" [3] has been offered twice a year since 2003 (Box 2). The number of participants is limited to 25 because of the hands-on and interactive nature of the learning. The course grew out of the authors' need to train their residents and fellows to be able to initiate recordings, to be aware of potential artifacts, and to recognize major abnormalities, with access by phone to advice from more experienced users. The fact that Bristol has been a major recruiting center for trials of therapeutic hypothermia and is a referral center for neonatal neurosurgery lay behind the need to provide continuous EEG 24 hours a day [4].

The participants receive course learning materials with copies of most of the teaching slides at the start of the day, and are given a certificate of completion at the end of the course.

The objectives of this course are to enable staff with little or no previous experience to initiate a continuous EEG recording, and to be aware of the limited, but important, information that it may provide in certain clinical situations.

Box 2. Curriculum for the Bristol 1-day course "Cerebral Function Monitoring and Neurophysiology for Neonatologists."

The morning consists of short lectures on:
1. The physiologic basis of EEG and the maturation of EEG with gestational age
   a) Impedance
   b) Physiological changes with waking/sleeping
   c) The concepts of continuity/discontinuity and interburst interval [5]
   d) Pathologic changes, including increased interburst interval, burst suppression, low-amplitude activity, and flat trace
   e) Characteristics of seizure activity on EEG
   f) Recognition of artifact, including muscle activity and electrical interference

2. The processing of the EEG by cerebral function monitors with normal appearances according to gestational age
   a) Waking/sleep cycles
   b) The grading system for term infants using pattern recognition: continuous normal voltage, discontinuous normal voltage, burst suppression, very low voltage, and flat trace [5]
   c) The grading system for term infants using voltage limits with normal upper margin of trace of more than 10 μV and lower margin of more than 5 μV [6]
   d) Appearances of seizures
   e) Appearances of artifact, including movement, procedure, and gasping

3. There then follows a practical session at which all four continuous EEG machines that are available in the United Kingdom—the Olympic CFM 6000 (Olympic Medical, Seattle, Washington), The BrainZ BRM2 (BrainZ Instruments, Auckland, Australia), the Nicolet One (Viasys, Madison, Wisconsin), and the Cerebral Function Analysis Monitor (CFAM4; RDM Consultants, Uckfield, United Kingdom)—are displayed and operated. Course participants are shown how to apply skin electrodes and are invited to apply them to each other on the frontotemporal skin with satisfactory impedance. A short recording of amplitude-integrated EEG (aEEG) is made using frontal electrodes with eyes closed and then with eyes open. Participants are shown how to insert and fix subdermal needle electrodes and practice inserting them into

a grapefruit. Archiving and accessing of recordings is demonstrated and the ability to sample EEG within a cerebral function monitor (CFM) recording is shown.

4. After lunch, there is a short lecture on the concept of cortical evoked potentials and the limited clinical application is described.

5. Five illustrative cases are presented, illustrating how continuous EEG aided clinical management. These include a case of perinatal asphyxia at term where the burst suppression EEG was part of the inclusion criteria for a hypothermia trial; an infant who had perinatal asphyxia where the initial EEG was normal, excluding hypoxic-ischemic encephalopathy (HIE) to the great relief of the parents; a preterm infant who had ventricular dilatation who was shown to have extremely abnormal slow seizures that led to an MRI showing lissencephaly; a term infant who had perinatal asphyxia where the initial burst suppression pattern at 3 hours of age had normalized by 12 hours, which changed the prognosis from 75% poor outcome to a probably good outcome; and a term infant whose ambiguous movements were difficult to interpret, but the EEG showed definite seizures, which led to a confident decision to start anticonvulsant therapy.

6. The next session is role-play. It is an important clinical skill of the neonatologist to explain to parents what investigations mean to their infant, because the neurophysiologist usually does not tell the parents what an EEG means. The participants are divided into three groups of eight to nine, and each group is given a clinical scenario with a corresponding CFM/EEG recording. The group's task is to decide the medical assessment and significance of the CFM trace, and how they should be explained to the baby's parent. One member of each group is selected or volunteers to role-play this in a plenary session, explaining to an actor parent who reacts with appropriate questions, anxiety, fear, relief, or incomprehension according to the explanation. The role-play session has received good feedback from the participants who recognize the importance of the skill and that medical knowledge is not all that is required.

7. The final session of the course is a test with 10 CFM/EEG traces with specific questions on the findings. This is marked, and feedback on the correct answers is given.

The authors teach these clinical indications for continuous EEG in the neonatal ICU:

Full-term infants who have marked acidosis at birth (pH < 7.0 or base deficit ≥ 16) or 5-minute Apgar scores of 5 or less

Full-term infants with lesser evidence of perinatal asphyxia but who have abnormal neurologic findings after birth, such as markedly abnormal tone or responsiveness

Infants of any gestation with abnormal movements that raise suspicion of seizure activity

Severe apnea, especially if repeated

Critically ill infants receiving muscle relaxants to facilitate ventilation

Additional indications may include preterm infants with grade III and IV intraventricular hemorrhage [7], preterm infants with birth weights of less than 750 g during the first 72 hours, infants who have congenital heart disease that is severe enough to require surgical intervention in the neonatal period (before and after surgery) [8], and infants before, during, and after extracorporeal membrane oxygenation [9]. It also has been suggested that physiologic cycling on continuous EEG could help to time handling and care disturbances to avoid disturbing quiet sleep [10–12].

Skin electrodes versus subdermal needle electrodes

In the authors' teaching they recommend the routine use of subdermal needle electrodes in critically ill infants where speed is important and neonatal staff have many other urgent clinical tasks. It usually takes no more than 5 minutes to have three needle electrodes in place and with a single-channel EEG running. The authors never have to shave the hair to get needle electrodes to function. The authors have kept needle electrodes in place for up to 5 days and never have had an infection. The authors' nursing staffs have observed needle electrodes and skin electrodes, and consistently prefer needle electrodes in critical care, believing that there is far less disturbance to the infant. In low-dependency situations where the infant is not critically ill and there is time, skin electrodes are preferred by some of the authors' staff, although the time that is required to achieve low impedance and the prolonged disturbance to the infant persuade some to use needle electrodes. Needle electrodes are not readily available for all brands of neonatal EEG monitors, so this issue should be reviewed carefully before making a decision on which type of monitor is purchased.

Single-channel electroencephalography may not be adequate

There are clinical situations in which a single-channel amplitude-integrated EEG (aEEG) is not adequate. This is particularly true when a unilateral cerebral lesion, such as middle cerebral artery infarction, is confirmed or is likely on clinical grounds. If clinical history or observation strongly

A

Neonatal Continuous EEG Monitoring Report Sheet

Name_____ Sex: M F DOB _____ GA _____ Birthweight _____

Hospital No_____ Electrode type: needle gel Monitor type _____

Indication for recording: _____

Date and time period						
Lower margin μvolt						
Upper margin μvolt						
Predominant pattern						
Quiet/active cycling						
Seizures						
Impedance						
Artifact?						

Medications _____

Interventions _____

Clinical status – Neuro _____

Respiratory _____

Comments _____

Signature/name _____

Fig. 1. (*A*) Neonatal continuous EEG monitoring report sheet. Time period is user-defined; use a separate period for each distinct change in background activity. All medications (anticonvulsants and otherwise) should be noted, as well as any interventions that might have affected the tracing. Note values for each hemisphere if two channels used and there is asymmetry, and use comments section to note any other asymmetric findings. *Predominant pattern coding:* CNV, continuous normal voltage; D, discontinuous; BS+, ≥100 bursts/h; BS−, <100 bursts/h; CLV, continuous low voltage; I, Inactive. Quiet/active cycling: N, not present; T, transitional; Y, yes. Seizure coding: A, absent; P, present (list number); S, status epilecticus. (*Adapted from* Hellstrom-Westas L, Rosen I, de Vries LS, et al. EEG classification and integration in preterm and term infants. NeoReviews 2006;7:e76–87). (*B*) Continuous, with cycling. (*C*) Continuous, no cycling. (*D*) Discontinuous pattern. (*E*) Burst suppression with more than 100 bursts/h. (*F*) Burst-suppression with less than 100 bursts/h. (*G*) Continuous low voltage less than 10 μV. (*H*) Inactive (flat) trace less than 5μV. (*I*) Seizures (diagnosis requires EEG confirmation) showing gradual build-up, then decline in amplitude of repetitive rhythmic spikes or sharp waves with duration of at least 10 seconds. (*J*) Repeated seizures (at least two seizures/h). (*K*) Status epilecticus (continuous seizures ≥30 minutes).

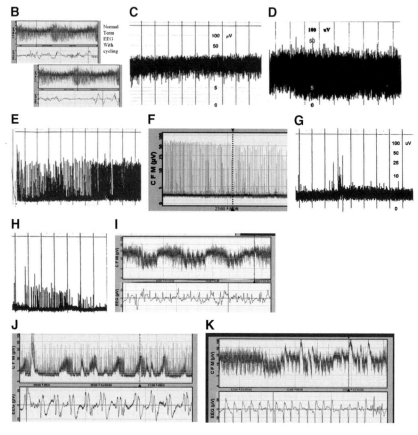

Fig. 1 (*continued*)

suggests focal seizures, then two or more channels are essential to exclude electrical seizures reliably. If the neonatal unit has an aEEG machine with only one channel then the clinical neurophysiology department will need to be involved.

Reporting of continuous electroencephalography for clinical purposes

Although neonatal EEG has been reported in different ways in different centers, the First International Conference on Neonatal Brain Monitoring in Florida in January 2006 showed that there is an emerging common language that describes the limited number of findings in neonatal EEG that have direct clinical significance.

The first widely used system for reporting aEEG recordings in newborns was reported by al Naqeeb and colleagues in 1999 [6]. This system classified recordings as "normal", "moderately abnormal," or "suppressed" on the basis of the upper and lower voltage margins of aEEG activity, and was shown to be highly predictive of outcome when used in term or near-term infants who had encephalopathy.

A system for scoring aEEG tracings in preterm infants was reported by Burdjalov and colleagues in 2003 [13]. By evaluating sleep-wake cycling, continuity of the tracing, and width of the band of aEEG activity, they were able to define normal values for various gestational ages.

Subsequently, Hellstrom-Westas and colleagues incorporated elements from both systems, as well as additional information about burst-suppression and seizure activity, to produce the most current definitions as described in their review earlier this year [5]. It is these definitions that the authors use in their suggested clinical report document shown in Fig. 1.

Interpreting the continuous EEG happens at various levels. There is the bedside observation by the baby's nurse and by medical staff in the immediate vicinity who may well have other immediate tasks. The nurse has an important role in marking events on the EEG monitor if the baby is handled, has a procedure, or shows abnormal movements. It also is important for the nurse to be aware that electrodes may become loose, and that this is revealed by an increase in impedance. The nurse needs to inform a neonatologist if seizure activity is suspected, or if there is a change on the monitor. In any case, if there has been a good clinical reason to record EEG, it is good practice in a neonatal ICU for a neonatologist to look at the monitor screen every few hours even if nothing has been reported.

The authors write a report every 24 hours using the format shown in Fig. 1. The reporter is asked to consider the recording in six 4-hour epochs, but, if necessary, a period of 6 hours could be divided into six 1-hour epochs. Impedance is checked and artifact considered first. The reporter is asked specifically to describe the average lower margin and upper margin voltage and to estimate burst frequency if the trace is discontinuous. The predominant pattern from one of six categories is allocated for each epoch. The presence of seizures is noted and whether they are repetitive or status. Presence of sleep/wake cycling is described, and any changes following medications and interventions (eg, cooling) are noted.

Quality control of reporting of continuous electroencephalography

If the EEG has been reported by a neonatologist who has taken the authors' course but has less than 1 year's experience with neonatal EEG, the recording is reviewed and finally signed off by a neonatologist with more experience. The authors find it good practice to have a meeting (or sit-down neonatal neurology rounds) once a week where the week's EEG recordings can be shown, each with the clinical story and neuroimaging. This acts as a final review and also has considerable educational value.

Although each recording is automatically filed on the hard disc of the equipment, it is important to have a separate copy on a CD or memory disc.

Paper record of significant findings and database for audit

It is useful to print out EEG findings that have important clinical significance and file these in the infant's medical chart. This means that one has a paper record in case all of the computers crash. It also is important to have a database containing a summary of the EEG findings together with minimal patient details. This approach is essential for audit of EEG recording activity, for reviewing diagnostic or clinical groups of patients, and for annual reports.

Are nationally recognized qualifications in continuous neonatal electroencephalography necessary?

There is the potential for inappropriate clinical decisions if continuous EEG is misinterpreted, particularly if artifact is not recognized. Thus, there is an argument for having recognized standards of competence, or a "driver's license." The bureaucracy and cost that are involved in national or international certification would not be justified in the authors' view, however. As an analogy, mechanical ventilation is capable of considerably more abuse to babies than is EEG, but competence with ventilation generally is assessed locally rather than nationally. All large neonatal ICUs have developed their own internal training schemes for training, retraining, and competency testing of medical and nursing staff with the locally used ventilators. In addition, there are many national and international courses and conferences where advanced training in ventilation is available. High-frequency oscillation is a good example where a combination of international, national, and local teaching has produced competence without national licensing of "oscillator drivers." Thus, the authors would prefer to see the development of competence in continuous neonatal EEG follow the oscillatory ventilation model, rather than to have the technique limited strictly to board-certified neurophysiologists. Because of the requirement to keep recordings, neonatal staff must be aware that interpretations of continuous EEG may be reassessed. The wise neonatologist will be aware of her/his limitations, should be cautious about drawing conclusions from EEGs that are at variance with the rest of the clinical picture, and be willing to seek advice from an experienced colleague, using fax or e-mail to transmit the findings rapidly to another center. Such informal discussion about difficult EEGs may be easier in European countries because there are no fees charged for neonatal continuous EEG.

Involvement of industry in training?

There can be advantages to having equipment manufacturers supporting courses, in that demonstration equipment can be brought to the course venue and technical questions about a particular hardware or software may be answerable by specialist staff from the company. It is important that a course is not an advertisement for a particular company's products, however. In our experience, national and international courses must seek to have all relevant manufacturers taking part so that there is a fair opportunity for course delegates to see the whole range of technical possibilities and approaches. A local course for staff from one institution, however, can concentrate on the equipment that is available in that institution.

References

[1] Svenningsen NW, Blennow G, Lindroth M, et al. Brain-orientated intensive care treatment in severe neonatal asphyxia. Effects of phenobarbitone protection. Arch Dis Child 1982; 57(3):176–83.

[2] Hellstrom-Westas L, deVries LS, Rosen I. An atlas of amplitude-integrated EEGs in the newborn. London: Parthenon; 2003.

[3] A one-day course—Cerebral function monitoring and neurophysiology for neonatologists. Available at: http://www.neonatalneurology.org.uk/neurophysPoster.htm. Accessed July 11, 2006.

[4] Gluckman PD, Wyatt JS, Azzopardi D, et al. Selective head cooling with mild systemic hypothermia after neonatal encephalopathy: multicentre randomised trial. Lancet 2005; 365(9460):663–70.

[5] Hellstrom-Westas L, Rosen I, de Vries LS, et al. Amplitude-integrated EEG classification and integration in preterm and term infants. NeoReviews 2006;7:e76–87.

[6] al Naqeeb N, Edwards AD, Cowan FM, et al. Assessment of neonatal encephalopathy by amplitude-integrated electroencephalography. Pediatrics 1999;103(6 Pt 1):1263–71.

[7] Hellstrom-Westas L, Klette H, Thorngren-Jerneck K, et al. Early prediction of outcome with aEEG in preterm infants with large intraventricular hemorrhages. Neuropediatrics 2001; 32(6):319–24.

[8] Gaynor JW, Jarvik GP, Bernbaum J, et al. The relationship of postoperative electrographic seizures to neurodevelopmental outcome at 1 year of age after neonatal and infant cardiac surgery. J Thorac Cardiovasc Surg 2006;131(1):181–8.

[9] Gannon CM, Kornhauser MS, Gross GW, et al. When combined, early bedside head ultrasound and electroencephalography predict abnormal computerized tomography or magnetic resonance brain images obtained after extracorporeal membrane oxygenation treatment. J Perinatol 2001;21(7):451–5.

[10] Morelius E, Hellstrom-Westas L, Carlen C, et al. Is a nappy change stressful to neonates? Early Hum Dev 2006 Feb 26 [epub ahead of print].

[11] Westrup B, Hellstrom-Westas L, Stjernqvist K, et al. No indications of increased quiet sleep in infants receiving care based on the newborn individualized developmental care and assessment program (NIDCAP). Acta Paediatr 2002;91(3):318–22.

[12] Hellstrom-Westas L, Inghammar M, Isaksson K, et al. Short-term effects of incubator covers on quiet sleep in stable premature infants. Acta Paediatr 2001;90(9):1004–8.

[13] Burdjalov VF, Baumgart S, Spitzer AR. Cerebral function monitoring: a new scoring system for the evaluation of brain maturation in neonates. Pediatrics 2003;112(4):855–61.

CLINICS IN
PERINATOLOGY

Clin Perinatol 33 (2006) 679–691

High-Density Electroencephalogram Monitoring in the Neonate

William P. Fifer, PhD[a,b,*], Philip G. Grieve, PhD[c],
Jillian Grose-Fifer, PhD[d], Joseph R. Isler, PhD[c],
Dana Byrd, PhD[e]

[a]*College of Physicians and Surgeons, Columbia University, 630 West 168th Street,
New York, NY 10032, USA*
[b]*Sackler Institute of Developmental Psychobiology, New York State Psychiatric Institute,
1051 Riverside Drive, Unit 40, New York, NY, 10032, USA*
[c]*Division of Neonatology, College of Physicians and Surgeons, Columbia University,
630 West 168th Street, New York, NY 10032, USA*
[d]*Division of Perinatology, College of Physicians and Surgeons, Columbia University,
630 West 168th Street, New York, NY 10032, USA*
[e]*Division of Developmental Psychobiology, Department of Psychiatry,
College of Physicians and Surgeons, Columbia University, 630 West 168th Street,
New York, NY 10032, USA*

The electroencephalogram (EEG) is the electrical potential generated by brain neural activity, predominantly from the cerebral cortex. It is measurable over the entire scalp surface as a continuous measure or "field" [1]. Regional differences in the potential correspond to differential activity in different brain areas. Sensitive amplifiers measure potential (voltage) differences at a discrete set of electrode sites. Therefore, if an accurate topographical map is to be obtained, the measurement sites must be numerous and in close proximity. This requirement is similar to that for the number of pixels in an image displayed on a computer. If there are too few pixels, the image is blurry and distorted. Recent work has shown that at least 64 equally spaced leads are needed to cover the scalp in an adult and at least 128 in an infant to produce accurate plots of the EEG over the scalp. Infants benefit from more leads than adults, as their skulls are comparatively thin and thereby produce less spatial blurring of the EEG [2].

This work was supported by NIH grants HD 32774 and EB000266.
* Corresponding author.
E-mail address: wpf1@columbia.edu (W.P. Fifer).

Electroencephalogram recording reference requirements

The EEG represents differences in electrical potential (microvolts) at many locations on the scalp. This requires the use of a reference potential with respect to which all the electrode voltages are measured. Many body locations have been proposed as a good reference point to use: ears, neck, nose, and top of head, among others. None of these points are ideal, however, because they each have an electric potential of their own arising from conducted bioelectrical currents. The perfect reference point, the "point at infinity," corresponds to a reference that is infinitely distant from the head. This, of course, is only an abstract mathematical concept. However, the dense array EEG system can produce a reference, the average reference, which is close to this ideal [3]. The average reference represents the average electrical activity from all the recording sites; as the number of electrodes on the scalp increases, the average reference more closely approximates the ideal reference. More than 100 electrodes are needed to achieve this optimal recording reference [4].

Spontaneous or evoked potential electroencephalogram

EEG can be measured in response to a sensory stimulus or can be recorded spontaneously when a subject is not attending to any particular event. The spontaneous EEG has been traditionally used by neurologists to diagnose neurologic disease or impairment. Traditionally, neurologists scan the EEG waveforms by eye to assess whether patterns of waveforms appear abnormal [5]. However, as the number of electrodes increases, it becomes difficult to use conventional methods for assessment.

An evoked potential waveform is typically much smaller in amplitude than the background spontaneous EEG. But because the evoked potential activity is time-locked to the stimulus and the background EEG is random, if the stimulus is presented multiple times, then an averaged waveform can be constructed. These signal-averaged waveforms also form a potential field on the scalp and have a more accurate topographic representation when observed with the dense array system. Furthermore, the dense array EEG greatly enhances the accuracy of locating the underlying brain sources of the surface-recorded electrical activity.

Electroencephalogram functional brain connectivity

Perhaps the greatest benefit of the dense array system is the ability to accurately measure synchrony between EEG waveforms. EEG synchrony is the basis for functional brain connectivity [6]. The premise of this method is that if EEG waveforms measured at two locations are highly correlated over time, neural groups in the vicinity of each electrode must be pursuing related activities. The related activity indicates a neural connection between the measurement sites (eg, corticocortical connections), connections to a third site (eg, corticothalamic connections), or both. Functional brain connectivity can be assessed by computing the synchrony (correlation) of EEG waveforms collected at pairs of locations over the entire scalp. Functional electrocortical connectivity can thus be measured at rest or in response to a stimulus. It is important that synchrony be calculated for all frequency components in the EEG because brain behaviors are known to be different at different EEG frequencies [5]. The excellent time resolution of the EEG enables the synchrony measurements of high-frequency brain oscillations (eg, gamma band 50Hz). This assessment cannot be done by eye and requires the use of computer-driven Fourier analyses. The importance of gamma oscillations has recently been acknowledged as important in the binding of distributed activities of various brain regions. Synchrony measurements are highly influenced by the accuracy of the average reference and the spacing and number of scalp electrodes (Fig. 1) [7].

The brain processes information locally, and this information is combined across other brain regions. Thus, it is important to measure synchrony locally (from two closely spaced electrodes) and at long distances (two electrodes far apart). Local synchrony can be measured with electrodes as close as 1 cm apart. The thin skulls of infants afford even more accurate measurement of local synchrony as there is less spatial blurring than in adults [8]. High-density EEG is therefore essential for accurate synchrony measurement because it uses over 100 electrodes to give an accurate average reference and provides full scalp coverage with the required close (1 cm) spacing [3].

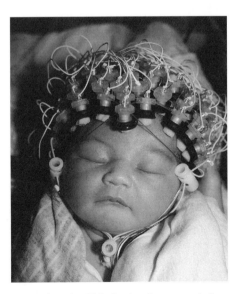

Fig. 1. A neonate undergoing high-density electroencephalogram recording.

High-density advantages

There are many practical issues that come into play in the clinical evaluation of the neonate. Of course a primary concern is patient safety, and one safety issue is risk of infection. High-density nets and caps, when used with high-impedance-tolerant amplifiers, reduce the risk of skin irritation and possible infection by eliminating the necessity of abrasion of the skin beneath electrode sites. High-impedance amplifiers allow these electrodes to have simple contact connection to the unabraded scalp, once any hair is pushed aside, using an electrolyte (saline or gel) solution preapplied to the electrodes. Unlike some single-site electrodes, however, high-density electrodes are not disposable. The recording caps/nets must be thoroughly disinfected after use. This is often true for all reusable medical equipment and is not a limitation in practice.

A second practical advantage of the high-density EEG system is the relative tolerance of the cap/net by the infant. The use of molding foam beneath the head and neck reduces scalp pressure points, which can arise as a consequence of the extensive electrode coverage, and can therefore extend the period of time the high-density net is tolerated by neonates to an hour or longer. Traditional EEG electrode application is time-consuming, especially if multiple electrodes are used, because each scalp area needs to be abraded to reduce skin impedance. In contrast, the high-density net can be quickly placed on the head, and data collection can begin in just a few minutes. The trade-off for rapid placement is less-than-exact placement of each electrode. Careful placement of the net allows for reasonable correlation with underlying brain areas, though this can differ slightly with the shape of the infant's head, especially for those neonates tested soon after vaginal delivery. This registration also requires additional time. Some high-density EEG systems, such as those manufactured by Electrical Geodesics, Inc. (EGI; www.egi.com), have developed spatial mapping systems for the instantaneous determination of absolute spatial coordinates of the electrodes.

One major benefit of high-density EEG collection is the flexibility of the off-line analyses. Data sets can be observed using a range of different reference points, allowing comparisons of average-referenced data to more traditionally recorded single-site clinical data or for comparing scalp locations of interest with other published data sets. The data can also be examined continuously as a clinical EEG recording or parsed into epochs, cleaned of artifact, and averaged to examine evoked potentials. For evoked potential analysis, the large number of electrodes over a given area of scalp provides the advantage of spatial averaging across adjacent electrodes. This approach affords improved signal-to-noise ratios, potentially allowing the recording of an evoked response averaged from few stimulus responses, as with infrequent/oddball stimuli or during multiple stages of recovery from anesthesia.

High-density EEG systems are expensive because they have a large number of amplifiers (one per lead). The increased amount of digital data is easily stored with the inexpensive hard drives currently available, however. Of greater concern is the application time for a large number of leads to the subject's scalp. Two systems are currently in vogue—one with preamplifiers located at the scalp electrode site, which provides superior artifact rejection but requires each electrode scalp site to be individually prepared with gel, and another that uses sponge electrodes wetted with an electrolyte (NaCl or KCl) that are pressed to the scalp by an elastic tension structure. The latter system is more rapidly applied to the patient (a few minutes compared with 30 minutes) but is more sensitive to movement artifact and is subject to electrodes drying out in long studies. The authors have successfully used the sponge system for intra-operating-room recording for 4 to 6 hours, however, if the electrodes are covered with plastic wrap to decrease evaporation. The choice of systems depends, ultimately, on the requirements of the user.

Evoked potentials

An evoked potential (EP) is the averaged electrical activity recorded from the scalp (EEG) that is elicited in response to a stimulus. Auditory, visual, and somatosensory stimuli have been used from infancy to adulthood as a means to study neural integrity and its development in various modalities. Functionality and maturity may be assessed at different hierarchical levels of the nervous system using evoked potential technology. For example, early components in the auditory-evoked potential (< 15 ms in the adult) reflect brainstem activity, whereas later slow waves arise from cortical structures that process auditory information.

Neonatal EPs share some basic characteristics across sensory modalities: they are simple waveforms with fewer components than adult EPs. The appearance, timing and amplitude of the waveform are specific to the modality and physical attributes of the stimulus. The timing (latency) of the EP waves, which reflect neural maturity, integrity, and myelination of sensory systems, are of long latencies. Long interstimulus intervals are required during the neonatal period to prevent amplitude reduction caused by fatigue. Waveform complexity and latencies vary as a function of gestational age.

Flash visual-evoked potentials

A bright flash of light has been a popular stimulus to record visual-evoked potentials (VEPs) from uncooperative subjects. Consequently, there is an extensive literature regarding responses from full-term and preterm neonates and their subsequent development throughout infancy. The earliest gestational age at which a flash VEP has been recorded is 24 weeks' gestational age (GA), and the most consistent feature in newborns of less than 36 weeks' GA is a negative wave (N3), which has a peak latency of 300 ms or more [9–10]. At 36 weeks' GA, a preceding positive wave (P2) is typically present at about 200 ms. A major advantage of using a flash is that it is bright enough to elicit a response through closed eyelids and can therefore, in theory, be used across different sleep states. However, sleep state can affect morphology and latency of the VEP [11–15], and the International Society of Clinical Electrophysiology and Vision (ISCEV) advises that recording should be performed only when the infant is behaviorally alert. Because alertness is infrequent and short-lived during the neonatal period, the use of an electrode recording system such as the EGI cap maximizes the likelihood of optimal recording because it can be applied quickly, is well tolerated, and can remain in place for long periods. The flash elicits a large amplitude response that is easily recordable with a minimum of averaging. Once the newborn is awake and quiet, it takes only a few minutes to record four runs of 30 flashes. A major advantage of using a high-density EEG system is that raw EEG from the whole head is always observable, and this information, coupled with behavioral observation, gives an accurate indication of the behavioral state of the infant. Quiet sleep has the greatest impact on the recording of the neonatal VEP; amplitudes are diminished (P2 sometimes absent) and latencies are longer than normal. An assessment of behavioral state is essential in the interpretation of the EP because an abnormal waveform is defined by a lack of components or components of longer than standard latency. Repeated runs are also useful in evaluating whether abnormal VEPs may be due to low arousal, as increased variability is common when the infant is not alert.

Clinical application of evoked potentials

Brainstem auditory-evoked potentials (BAEPs) are commonly used in neonatal auditory screening, and VEPs, often in conjunction with electroretinogram recording, are useful in diagnosing visual dysfunction during infancy. EPs reflect the summed brain activity in response to a specific stimulus and can be recorded with great temporal accuracy (milliseconds). EP peak latency is highly sensitive to the pathology of demyelination, and it is therefore presumed that the long latency components recorded during the neonatal period reflect the relative lack of myelination within the geniculo-localcarine tract; by 32 weeks, GA myelination is prechiasmal, and by 37 weeks, it has reached the optic tract. Further increases in myelination have a much longer time course [16]. Despite that the VEP is a potentially sensitive tool in evaluating CNS function, it is not widely capitalized on in clinical practice. Several studies have validated VEP recording in predicting neurodevelopmental outcome in high-risk term infants [17–19]. Controversy exists, however, over the prognostic viability of VEP in preterm infants [20]. Shepherd and colleagues [21] showed that a normal VEP recorded during the first few weeks of preterm life had limited predictive value, though others disagree [22]. Despite these differences, some consistencies emerged across studies, and reliability is enhanced by serial recordings at different ages (in preterm infants, recording at term is often useful). Severely abnormal (absent) VEPs have reliably shown to have severe neurodevelopmental consequences, commonly death or CP [21,23]. Combining information from VEPs and SSEPs improves predictability considerably [18].

Advantages of high density with event-related recordings

The amplitude of the neonatal flash VEP is largest over the occipital cortex, and many have used small numbers of recording electrodes (often one or two around the occiput) to successfully record the response [12]. However, waveform morphology and latencies can vary considerably over small distances (2 cm) and may be crucial in deciding whether a VEP falls within normal limits [22]. The large number of recording electrodes afforded by the high-density EEG system allows a large area of cortex to be sampled. Consequently, this eliminates the need for surface landmarks traditionally used to infer the position of underlying cortical areas, which may be advantageous if neonatal and adult brain anatomy differ in relation to these landmarks. An electrode array that adequately samples the occipital cortex activity enhances the clinical usefulness of the VEP by eliminating the recording of falsely abnormal VEPs caused by suboptimal electrode placement.

The maturational changes in the EP have been attributed to several possible factors, including dendritic branching in layer V of visual cortex, synaptogenesis, and myelination in the visual cortex. However, others have suggested that the neonatal vision may be subcortically mediated, which would suggest that the immature VEP may reflect extrageniculocalcarine activity [24–28]. A further advantage of the high-density EEG system affords better localization of intracranial generators of evoked potentials, which may give better indications of the sources of the neonatal components.

Alternative analyses of visual-evoked potentials with high density

A limitation of the traditional averaging technique used for recording evoked potentials is that it requires the neural response to be time-locked to the stimulus; if there is any "jitter" (variable latency) in the neural response, then the response will be underestimated when averaging over repeated stimuli. The earliest ERP components (corresponding to responses from early sensory processing) are the most consistently reproducible components in amplitude and latency [29]. Presumably, higher-level or more widespread aspects of the response are not as time-locked to the stimulus as the earlier lower-level aspects of the response and are therefore not as easily evaluated. Not surprisingly, only early evoked potential components (BAEP, SSEP, and VEP) been found to have clinical use. However, alternative analysis techniques could provide measures of later ERP components that are not as rigidly time-locked as the early sensory components.

To illustrate the use of alternative ERP analyses, the authors present results of an infant study. In the laboratory, visual-evoked potentials to a flash stimulus were recorded from 19 newborn infants using a high-density EEG system (EGI). Data were analyzed using both the traditional averaged waveform approach and an alternative approach, cross-spectral analysis. Typical infant VEPs, with a positive component with a latency of about 200 ms, were observed in most infants with movement free trials. However, in some cases a clear VEP component was not seen. A striking example of the possibilities for alternative ERP measures is shown in Fig. 2. Here, results for the same VEP experiment performed in two infants are shown. One infant (top) showed a classic VEP component as a large positive peak around 200 ms poststimulus in posterior electrodes. The same procedure in the other infant (bottom) failed to elicit a clear VEP component. In contrast, for both infants, cross-spectral amplitudes in the beta frequency range (23 Hz) show clear responses over posterior electrodes at the time of VEP latency.

Synchrony measures

The cross-spectrum measures the magnitude of phase locking or synchrony between electrode pairs at a given frequency [30]. Other algorithms that measure synchrony, such as coherence (the cross-spectrum normalized by power) and phase synchronization (circular variance of the phase difference between two signals), can also be used to construct a measure of synchrony response to a given stimulus and are being investigated in the authors' laboratory. As mentioned previously, synchrony is a fundamental brain mechanism that acts across a wide range of spatial and temporal scales, with important roles in development, local functionality, perceptual binding, and memory [31]. Thus, methods of ERP analysis that explicitly measure synchrony within and between brain regions offer another important measurement of neural function. Synchronization may occur at high EEG frequencies, but because of their low amplitude, they make minimal contributions to the averaged waveform. Consequently, these alternative methods of analysis offer new insights into brain development.

Shown on the right side of Fig. 2 is the difference between the cross-spectrum at VEP latency (128–256 ms) and cross-spectrum averaged across the baseline interval, for 23Hz. This variation can be considered to be the cross-spectral response to the stimulus at 128 to 256 ms and 23 Hz. The cross-spectral responses at 15, 30, and 38 Hz also showed enhanced synchrony at this VEP latency, but the response was clearest at 23 Hz. With the electrical geodesics numbering scheme for the electrode net used in these experiments, electrodes that are spatially contiguous are not always neighbors in the cross-spectrum matrix. This accounts for the appearance of stripes within the matrices.

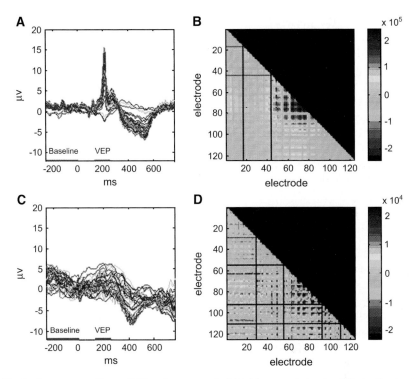

Fig. 2. Average waveforms (*left*) and cross-spectral (*right*) response to visual flash stimulus in newborn infants. Results for a block of 30 flashes for two infants are shown. The first infant (*top row*) showed a clear visual-evoked potential (VEP) component with a latency of about 200 ms and amplitude of 5–15 uV (*A*). Enhanced synchrony at VEP latency is located primarily over occipital regions (electrodes 60–90) (*B*). A second infant (*bottom row*) showed little evidence of the VEP component in the averaged waveforms (*C*). Despite the greater variance in the averaged waveforms and lack of a clear VEP component, enhanced synchrony at VEP latency over occipital regions is clearly evident in the cross-spectrum in the second infant (*D*). Methods: Thirty 100-ms light flashes 3 s apart were delivered to each infant. Data were sampled at 1000 Hz and segmented into 1024-ms windows about the time of flash onset, with 256 ms before flash and 768 ms after flash. Averaged waveforms were included if two-thirds of trials passed artifact rejection criteria (SD < 15 uV, absolute excursions < 150 uV.). Electrodes with data rejected by conservative artifact rejection schemes were filled with minimum values and appear as blue stripes. Cross-spectra were calculated at 23 Hz by averaging over trials for nonoverlapping 128-ms segments, yielding two estimates before stimulus (to assess the baseline cross-spectrum) and six estimates poststimulus (to characterize evolution of the cross-spectral response).

As can be seen in the bottom left of Fig. 2, the variance is greater in the waveforms of the second infant. This difference would reflect a lower signal-to-noise ratio if one considers the stimulus-elicited response to be the signal and the background EEG to be the noise. If that were the case, a much larger number of trials (there were 60–90 stimuli in these experiments) would have succeeded in eliciting the VEP component in the second infant.

Alternatively, the presence of a significant cross-spectral measure for the second infant in the absence of an averaged VEP component could be explained if local synchrony was enhanced, but the full set of conditions required to generate the VEP component did not occur. In either case, local synchrony would be a more robust measure of visual response to flash in visual cortex.

These results suggest that enhanced posterior high-frequency synchrony is a measure of neural response in visual cortex that provides useful information in addition to the classic VEP waveform component. Frequency-dependent synchrony may prove to be an even more sensitive and specific measure of neural response than the time-domain-averaged waveform.

Response to sensory novelty

An experimental paradigm known to elicit activity in brain areas beyond primary sensory areas is called the oddball paradigm. In this paradigm, a train of stimuli are presented, wherein the most frequent (standards) are invariably the same, and the less frequent (nonstandards) are "oddballs." The oddballs may be all the same (deviants) or individually unique (novels). For example, a sound train may consist of a random sequence of 90% standard 1000 Hz tones and 10% deviant 1300 Hz tones (in the auditory modality the oddballs may differ in frequency, intensity, or duration). The resulting ERP will show the deviant response to differ from the standard response. The oddball waveform (polarity, peak/trough latencies, and integrated power) varies with experimental design. When sounds are unattended, the difference between deviant and standard waveforms is called mismatch negativity (MMN). The MMN component is considered to correspond to an automatic, preattentive change detection mechanism to sounds, primarily involving the auditory cortex. The MMN can be elicited in neonates and is particularly suited for infant ERP studies because it is elicited in the absence of attention [32]. Since its discovery in the 1970s, its clinical usefulness has also been extensively explored [33]. Change detection involves sensory discrimination and short-term sensory memory; therefore, MMN abnormalities in infants and children are correlated with, and may be predictive of, impairment in related cognitive skills [34–36].

Electroencephalogram during neonatal learning

The ability to demonstrate learning during the neonatal period has been recognized for some time. Traditional EEG systems and limited analytical algorithms, however, have precluded systematic investigation of coincident brain activity during behavioral learning tasks. EEG recordings during sequences of contingent (associated) stimuli may provide a window into investigating distributed neural systems. The authors are currently conducting studies using high-density EEG recordings to examine the cerebellar-cortical circuitry abnormalities that have been implicated in many developmental disorders, such as autism and cerebellar-mediated cerebral palsy, which occurs in a subset of premature infants. To probe this neural circuitry, high-density EEG from neonates during delay eye-blink conditioning has been recorded, a form of conditioning that is known from decades of animal research to rely on cerebellar-cortical connections (see Fig. 3). These high-density scalp recordings have been used not only for the examination of EEG responses to stimuli but also for observation of a behavioral response.

Recording of high-sampling rate, high-density (full-scalp coverage) EEG from newborn infants during conditioning allows for the decomposition of the EEG signal across the scalp to isolate and ignore components caused by electrical noise present in the unshielded newborn nursery environment and from infant movement. This approach has allowed us to determine the presence of a conditioned blink response, even when the eyes are closed during sleep. The frontal scalp distribution and rapid onset shape of a component waveform signals the onset of a conditioned blink caused by the electrical signal generated by the retina changing position as the eye rolls upward, with and without observable blinks.

Additionally, independent components analysis (ICA) of the high-density data is used to remove artifacts to uncover a conditioning-generated event-related potential (ERP). This ERP, the contingent negative variation (CNV), has been shown in animal and human intracranial research to be elicited by the cerebellar-thalamocortical circuitry during conditioning. In summary, analytic techniques, including measures of synchrony, coupling,

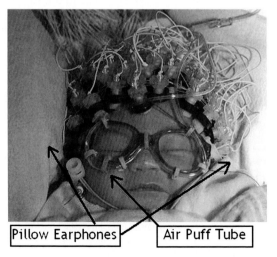

Fig. 3. Newborn infant instrumented with high-density electroencephalogram net for eye-blink conditioning task that requires multiple pairings of sound with simultaneous air puffs.

and spectral evolution, applied in addition to standard averaged-waveform analysis should lead to the development of new clinical and diagnostic tools for assessing the integrity of cortical function in infants.

Summary

High-density EEG has emerged as a viable tool for noninvasive analysis of neonatal brain function. This minimal risk technology offers a promising new direction for EEG measurement of brain activity in neonatal research and clinical practice. The potential advantages may emerge during measurement of both spontaneous and evoked activity. The analysis of waveforms observed with the dense array system may aid in localizing the source of scalp potentials. Analysis of synchrony and coherence from multiple electrodes may offer insight into the development of brain connectivity and may afford analysis of acute responses to environmental conditions as well as early diagnosis of abnormal neurologic trajectories in the high-risk infant.

References

[1] Physiological basis of EEG. In: Ebersole JS, Pedley TA, editors. Current practice of clinical electroencephalography. 3rd edition. Philadelphia: Lippincott Williams & Wilkins; 1997. p. 107–38.
[2] Grieve PG, Emerson RG, Isler JR, et al. Quantitative analysis of spatial sampling error in the infant and adult electroencephalogram. Neuroimage 2004;21(4):1260–74.
[3] Junghofer M, Elbert T, Tucker DM, et al. The polar average reference effect: a bias in estimating the head surface integral in EEG recording. Clin Neurophysiol 1999;110(6):1149–55.
[4] Nunez P, editor. Electric fields of the brain. New York: Oxford University Press; 1981.
[5] Fingelkurts AA, Fingelkurts AA, Kahkonen S. Functional connectivity in the brain—is it an elusive concept? Neurosci Biobehav Rev 2005;28(8):827–36.
[6] Nunez PL, Silberstein RB, Shi Z, et al. EEG coherency II: experimental comparisons of multiple measures. Clin Neurophysiol 1999;110(3):469–86.
[7] Nunez PL, Srinivasan R, Westdorp AF, et al. EEG coherency. I: Statistics, reference electrode, volume conduction, Laplacians, cortical imaging, and interpretation at multiple scales. Electroencephalogr Clin Neurophysiol 1997;103(5):499–515.
[8] Grieve PG, Emerson RG, Fifer WP, et al. Spatial correlation of the infant and adult electroencephalogram. Clin Neurophysiol 2003;114(9):1594–608.
[9] Taylor MJ, Menzies R, MacMillan LJ, et al. VEPs in normal full-term and premature neonates: longitudinal versus cross-sectional data. Electroencephalogr Clin Neurophysiol 1987; 68(1):20–7.
[10] Chin KC, Taylor MJ, Menzies R, et al. Development of visual evoked potentials in neonates. A study using light emitting diode goggles. Arch Dis Child 1985;60(12):1166–8.
[11] Lodge A, Armigton JC, Barnet AB, et al. Newborn infants' electroretinograms and evoked electroencephalographic responses to orange and white light. Child Dev 1969;40(1):267–93.
[12] Umezaki H, Morrell F. Developmental study of photic evoked responses in premature infants. Electroencephalogr Clin Neurophysiol 1970;28(1):55–63.
[13] Watanabe K, Iwase K, Hara K. Visual evoked responses during different phases of quiet sleep in pre-term infants. Neuropadiatrie 1973;4(4):427–33.

[14] Whyte HE, Pearce JM, Taylor MJ. Changes in the VEP in preterm neonates with arousal states, as assessed by EEG monitoring. Electroencephalogr Clin Neurophysiol 1987;68(3): 223–5.

[15] Grose J, Harding GFA, Wilton AY, et al. The maturation of the pattern-reversal VEP and flash ERG in pre-term infants. Clin Vis Sci 1989;4:239–46.

[16] Takayama S, Yamamoto M, Hashimoto K, et al. Immunohistochemical study on the developing optic nerves in human embryos and fetuses. Brain Dev 1991;13(5):307–12.

[17] Eken P, van Nieuwenhuizen O, van der Graaf Y, et al. Relation between neonatal cranial ultrasound abnormalities and cerebral visual impairment in infancy. Dev Med Child Neurol 1994;36(1):3–15.

[18] Taylor MJ, Murphy WJ, Whyte HE. Prognostic reliability of somatosensory and visual evoked potentials of asphyxiated term infants. Dev Med Child Neurol 1992;34(6):507–15.

[19] Muttitt SC, Taylor MJ, Kobayashi JS, et al. Serial visual evoked potentials and outcome in term birth asphyxia. Pediatr Neurol 1991;7(2):86–90.

[20] Ekert PG, Keenan NK, Whyte HE, et al. Visual evoked potentials for prediction of neurodevelopmental outcome in preterm infants. Biol Neonate 1997;71(3):148–55.

[21] Shepherd AJ, Saunders KJ, McCulloch DL, et al. Prognostic value of flash visual evoked potentials in preterm infants. Dev Med Child Neurol 1999;14(1):9–15.

[22] Kurtzberg D. Event-related potentials in the evaluation of high-risk infants. Ann N Y Acad Sci 1982;388:557–71.

[23] Whyte HE, Taylor MJ, Menzies R, et al. Prognostic utility of visual evoked potentials in term asphyxiated neonates. Pediatr Neurol 1986;2(4):220–3.

[24] Bronson G. The postnatal growth of visual capacity. Child Dev 1974;45(4):873–90.

[25] Scher MS, Richardson GA, Robles N, et al. Effects of prenatal substance exposure: altered maturation of visual evoked potentials. Pediatr Neurol 1998;18(3):236–43.

[26] Atkinson J. Human visual development over the first 6 months of life. A review and a hypothesis. Hum Neurobiol 1984;3(2):61–74.

[27] Kraemer M, Abrahamsson M, Sjostrom A. The neonatal development of the light flash visual evoked potential. Doc Ophthalmol 1999;99(1):21–39.

[28] Mushin J, Dubowitz LM, De Vries L, et al. The visual evoked potential in neonates with occipital lesions and holoprosencephaly. Behav Brain Res 1986;21(2):79–83.

[29] Nunez P, editor. Neocortical dynamics and human EEG rhythms. New York: Oxford University Press; 1995.

[30] Bendat JS, Piersol AG. Random data: analysis and measurement procedures. New York: John Wiley & Sons; 2000.

[31] Varela F, Lachaux JP, Rodriguez E, et al. The brainweb: phase synchronization and large-scale integration. Nat Rev Neurosci 2001;2(4):229–39.

[32] Naatanen R, Gaillard AW, Mantysalo S. Early selective-attention effect on evoked potential reinterpreted. Acta Psychol [Amst] 1978;42(4):313–29.

[33] Cheour M, Leppanen PH, Kraus N. Mismatch negativity (MMN) as a tool for investigating auditory discrimination and sensory memory in infants and children. Clin Neurophysiol 2000;111(1):4–16.

[34] Korpilahti P, Lang HA. Auditory ERP components and mismatch negativity in dysphasic children. Electroencephalogr Clin Neurophysiol 1994;91(4):256–64.

[35] Kemner C, Verbaten MN, Koelega HS, et al. Event-related brain potentials in children with attention-deficit and hyperactivity disorder: effects of stimulus deviancy and task relevance in the visual and auditory modality. Biol Psychiatry 1996;40(6):522–34.

[36] Tanaka M, Okubo O, Fuchigami T, et al. A study of mismatch negativity in newborns. Pediatr Int 2001;43(3):281–6.

ELSEVIER
SAUNDERS

Clin Perinatol 33 (2006) 693–706

CLINICS IN
PERINATOLOGY

Sleep and Brain Development

Stanley Graven, MD

*Department of Community and Family Health, USF College of Public Health,
13201 Bruce B. Downs Boulevard, MDC 56, Tampa, FL 33612, USA*

Before the mid-1930s, sleep was conceptualized as a time of brain rest. Sleep was believed to be a passive state with little brain activity. Researchers primarily were occupied with dreams and dream interpretation. Electroencephalogram (EEG) technology was basic and not well understood. In 1936, Loomis and colleagues [1] described the existence of different sleep states and changes in levels of brain activity during sleep that were based on different EEG wave patterns. This work signaled the beginning of scientific sleep research. It was not until 1953 that the pattern known as rapid eye movement (REM) sleep was described [2], followed soon by descriptions of sleep cycles in which periods of REM sleep were interspersed with periods of non-REM (NREM) sleep [3]. There were patterns to sleep, as well as levels or depth of sleep.

Terminology for sleep phases and levels was established in 1968 and continues to be used in studies of sleep states and their description [4]. The ability to relate EEG waves to specific structures and cell groupings was expanded vastly. This approach has advanced the understanding of sleep and its role in brain development and brain function; however, most of the research in sleep and early brain development does not appear in clinical journals.

Historically, researchers who are studying the field of sleep have been divided into two main groups. The first group of sleep studies was based on behaviors and behavioral sleep. Sleep states and timing were based on muscle movements, eyelid movements, heart rate patterns, and respiration. The second group of researchers based their studies on EEG patterns and changes. With technologic advancements, a third group of researchers is studying sleep using active brain-imaging techniques. Most events that are seen on brain imaging correlate with the EEG pattern, so that they relate to each other in time and state. Unfortunately, behavioral states do not

E-mail address: sgraven@hsc.usf.edu

correlate necessarily with the EEG changes and vary greatly between animal species. This article focuses on sleep stages and behaviors that are associated with characteristic EEG patterns.

Sleep development

The development of sleep patterns, the sequence of the appearance of sleep activities, and EEG patterns that are associated with sleep are species-specific. As a whole, none of the animal models, including primates, are closely aligned with the entire process of sleep development in humans. The specific patterns of physiologic changes, brain electrical activity, and developmental sequences are unique to human infants; however, there are individual components of sleep and sleep processes in animals that are useful in understanding human processes. Sequences and processes that are involved with sleep and sleep cycles are studied and described in animals because it is possible to provide great detail at a cellular level in an animal model. As an example, visual development and the role of sleep are well studied in several different animal models because the processes have many similarities to those found in human infants; however, the sequence for the development of REM and NREM sleep in humans is unique, with no precise replica in other animal species.

Human sleep is divided into two basic phases or types—REM and NREM—each with unique characteristics. Based on EEG patterns, NREM sleep is divided into four stages and REM sleep has one basic pattern [5]. Stage 1 NREM sleep is the transitional stage between sleep and wakefulness, often referred to as drowsy sleep. The EEG pattern is one of low amplitude theta wave activity. Stage 2 NREM sleep is the onset of true, quiet sleep with EEG spindles and K complexes as the primary characteristics [6]. Stage 2 sleep is presumed to play a role in learning and memory processing [6]. Stages 3 and 4 represent different "depths of sleep," but both are characterized by high-amplitude, synchronized slow waves. These waves are the main characteristic of stage 3 and 4 NREM sleep [7]. The human fetus or infant in stage 3 or 4 slow-wave sleep (deep or quiet sleep) has a regular heart rate, regular respirations, little or no eye movement, and the characteristic slow-wave sleep pattern on the EEG. This pattern is recognized easily and has been described well [5].

REM sleep (also called paradoxical sleep) is characterized by unique EEG activity, rapid eye movements, and atonia of the postural muscles; however, the atonia of the postural muscles is absent or intermittent until 2 to 3 months of age and is only intermittent in preterm infants [8]. Thus, the fetus in utero and the preterm infant after 28 to 30 weeks' gestation exhibit muscle movements in addition to REMs. The 3-month-old infant has persistent atonia of the postural muscles during REM sleep.

Between 20 and 28 weeks' gestational age, the human fetus has what is called indeterminate or "presleep." Motor and eyelid movements are unrelated to the irregular EEG patterns of the immature nervous system. None of the distinguishing EEG characteristics of REM or NREM sleep is present, and there are no active correlations with sleep; however, during this period of immature brain activity, several essential cellular events occur that are critical to the development of the neurosensory systems. These come from the initially random and then gradually more synchronous firing of the ganglion cells of the retina, auditory system, olfactory system, motor neurons, and sensory neurons of the spinal cord as well as other centers in the thalamus and brain stem. Firing of the ganglion cells is necessary for axon targeting and for achieving precise connections between the sensory organs and central processing centers. This process is needed for building early brain architecture. Fetuses and premature infants may have rest/activity cycles and ganglion cell activity before 28 weeks' gestation, but they exhibit none of the characteristic EEG changes that are associated with sleep states.

At approximately 28 weeks' gestational age, individual sleep patterns begin to emerge with the coordination of different sleep phenomena. These sleep patterns are discontinuous, with interspersed periods of little electrical activity. This finding is true for REM and NREM sleep periods. Discrete periods are characterized by REMs, alternating with periods of sustained quiet with few or no REMs [8,9]. It is believed that this change represents the start of true sleep cycles, with distinct but discontinuous REM and NREM sleep states. Periods of REM and NREM sleep are constant by 36 to 38 weeks' gestational age [9,10].

The appearance of distinct REM and NREM sleep states at 28 to 30 weeks' gestation is followed rapidly by the development of sleep cycles that have clear and distinct patterns of brain activity for each sleep state. In the initial sleep cycles, REM sleep predominates, and occupies most sleep time. As the infant approaches term, REM and NREM sleep become nearly equal and remain so for the early weeks of life. By 8 months of age, NREM sleep occupies nearly 80% of sleep time [10]. Between 28 weeks' gestational age and 3 months of age, there is a gradual and consistent change in the EEG wave pattern for REM and NREM sleep. There also is a major change in the motor activity at 3 months when consistent atonia of the postural muscles begins to occur with REM sleep. In the evolution and development of sleep cycles, REM and NREM sleep have distinct developmental processes from the immature patterns at 28 weeks' gestational age to mature, near adultlike patterns by 3 to 5 months of age [9,11]. These are illustrated well by Mizrahi and colleagues [12], Hellstrom-Westas and colleagues [13], and Clancy and colleagues [14].

Development of nonrapid eye movement sleep

NREM sleep first appears as a recognized sleep state around 28 weeks' gestational age. In early NREM sleep, the infant has evidence of a startle response and sucking, but few eyelid movements. Heart rate and respiration are regular. The initial EEG appears as an immature pattern with short bursts of activity and extended quiet intervals, called "trace discontinue" [12]. The tracing is characterized by generally slow waves in a burst-suppression pattern interspersed with extended periods of synchronous low voltage. This pattern gradually becomes more mature and continuous with periods of generalized voltage attenuation near term called "trace alternans." It is characterized by slow waves (delta bands: 0.5–4.0 Hz) and sleep spindles (7–14 Hz) by 5 to 8 months of age [12,14,15].

Development of rapid eye movement sleep

REM sleep, as a distinct sleep state, also begins at 28 weeks' gestational age. The first manifestations are movements of eyelids (REMs) and body movements, which include muscle twitches and gross movements of trunk and extremities. Muscle activity patterns alternate with atonia. By 2 to 3 months of age, the mature pattern of persistent atonia of the postural muscles becomes a regular characteristic of REM sleep [8,11]. REM sleep gradually matures into a continuous pattern, which reflects the neuronal activity of the neocortex, hippocampus, pons, thalamus, and midbrain reticular formation. Each cell group plays an important part in brain activity and development during REM sleep (Fig. 1) [16]. Patterns are near maturity by 5 to 8 months of age.

The neurology of rapid eye movement and nonrapid eye movement sleep

The human brain is active during sleep, especially REM sleep. Often, more brain activity occurs during REM sleep than in wakefulness. This

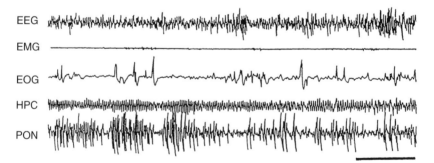

Fig. 1. REM sleep signal patterns. The EEG trace is from the cortex. The EMG shows the postural muscle atonia. The EOG shows eyelid movement. The HPC is the wave pattern from the hippocampus. The PON shows the P waves and spikes from the pons. (*Adapted from* Datta S. Avoidance task training potentiates phasic pontine-wave density in the rat: A mechanism for sleep-dependent plasticity. J Neurosci 2000;20:8607–13; with permission. ©2000 by the Society for Neuroscience.)

activity begins before the development of definable sleep states at approximately 28 weeks' gestational age. The transition from awake to sleep is not a passive process, but one that is stimulated actively by cell groups in the brain stem and thalamus. The awake state is stimulated and maintained by aminergic cell groups in the brain stem. REM sleep is stimulated actively by cholinergic cell groups. As the aminergic stimulation (awake state) wanes, NREM sleep begins. As the cholinergic stimulation increases, it reaches a point where sleep shifts from NREM sleep to REM sleep. Cell group patterns alternate in their activity level, which result in cycles of wakefulness, NREM sleep, and REM sleep [10,11]. There is no single control site or area. In each period of wakefulness, NREM and REM sleep are excited by distinct groups of cells in the brain stem. Each of the characteristic components of REM sleep is activated and regulated by different areas or cell groups [7]. The key neurologic components of REM sleep are listed in Table 1 [7].

During NREM sleep or slow-wave sleep, there is a deactivation process that produces slow waves and spindles that are characteristic of the NREM sleep EEG pattern. This process is controlled largely by the midbrain reticular formation that connects to the thalamus and from there to the cortex. The active balance between REM on and REM off stimulation is in the pontine reticular formation, and it is responsible for the sleep cycling [17].

Role of rapid eye movement and nonrapid eye movement sleep cycles in neurodevelopment

REM and NREM sleep cycling are essential for early neurosensory development, learning and memory, and preservation of brain plasticity for the life of the individual. In all animal studies in which these specific electrical

Table 1
The components of rapid eye movement sleep and the neurostructure responsible for the stimulation, waves, or oscillations

Component of REM sleep	Responsible brain structure
Desynchronized neocortical EEG pattern	Ponto-mesencephalic reticular formation (brainstem)
Postural muscle atonia	Locus coeruleus (brainstem)
REMs – Eye movement	Peri-abducens reticular formation (brainstem)
Hippocampus theta state	Nucleus reticularis
Theta waves or oscillations	Pontus oralis (Pons)
Pons	Pontine tegmentum (Pons)
P waves	
Pons	Pontine tegmentum, lateral geniculate
PGO spikes or waves	Nucleus and occipital cortex
Retinal waves	Ganglion cells of retina
Retinal ganglion cell stimulation	

waves or cell groups are blocked or the animals are deprived of REM sleep, permanent neurologic injury or failure of development results.

Neurosensory development

Two general categories of stimuli are essential for neurosensory development: activity-independent or endogenous stimuli, and activity-dependent or exogenous stimuli [12,18]. Endogenous stimuli arise from neurons within the neurosensory system and are unrelated to any outside sensory stimulation. In its earliest form, these are cell firings or discharges that begin soon after the ganglion cell or neuron has differentiated into a specific cell type. Repeated early discharges are essential for axon growth and targeting. As the human infant approaches 28 weeks' gestational age, various sensory and central brain systems begin propagation of synchronous waves and reciprocal oscillations that connect the sensory organs to the brainstem, thalamus, cortex, and other areas that are essential to neurosensory development. Synchronous ganglion cell waves and oscillations are independent of any outside stimulation. Patterns of endogenous stimulation occur only during REM sleep. Thus, REM sleep is essential to the process of endogenous stimulation and development of neurosensory systems [18,19].

The visual system is a well-studied example of this process [18,20]. Ganglion cells of the retina (Fig. 2) [21] begin frequent random firing before 28 weeks' gestational age as part of the growth and targeting of axons to the lateral geniculate nucleus (LGN). Thus, neurons of the LGN are stimulated to target axons to cells of the visual cortex. The same applies to the superior colliculus, which is essential for eye movement coordination. With maturation of the starburst amocrine cells of the retina (a special type of amocrine cell; see Fig. 2), the ganglion cells develop synchronous waves of activation [22]. Retinal ganglion cells stimulate synchronous waves to the cells of the LGN. LGN cells are stimulated by the PGO waves from the pons, which stimulates the cells of the visual cortex to form columns that are called ocular dominance columns. Ocular dominance columns are the essential framework for subsequent development of directional columns and other columns in the occipital lobe cortex that are needed for central vision reception. These latter columns develop in the visual cortex as a result of visual experience [20]. Retinal ganglion cell waves are essential to central visual system development and occur only as a function of REM sleep [22]. REM sleep deprivation results in failure of central visual development or disruption of structural and functional relationships of the central visual system.

Endogenous stimulation, which occurs as part of REM sleep in the preterm infant, plays a critical role in the initial development of sensory systems. Neurosensory systems and other systems that are dependent on endogenous stimulation that is associated with REM sleep in the preterm infant or fetus include:

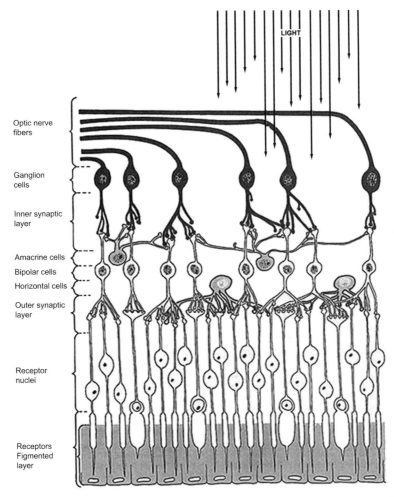

Fig. 2. The human retina. The five major cell types and three layers are shown. (*From* Palmer SE. Vision science: photons to phenomenology. Cambridge (MA): MIT Press; 1999. p. 30; with permission.)

Visual system
Auditory system
Somatesthetic (touch) system
Olfactory system
Limbic system, including amygdala, hypothalamus, and mammilary body involved with emotional experience
Hippocampus and the hippocampal cortical connections associated with learning and memory
Pons, thalamus, various reticular formations, and other centers in the brainstem and mid-brain

Development in all of these areas is delayed or disordered as a result of REM sleep deprivation or interference with the synchronous endogenous stimulation.

Following the initial development of endogenously stimulated neurosystems, these areas are readied for exogenous or activity-dependent stimulation. For the visual system, the need for visual experience occurs near term or 40 weeks' gestational age. Other systems listed above become responsive to exogenous stimulation as well as endogenous stimulation between 28 and 32 weeks' gestational age. Thus, the environment of the fetus in utero and of the preterm infant in the neonatal ICU (NICU) requires appropriate levels of specific types of exogenous neurosensory stimulation for healthy early brain development. This process does not include visual stimulation before term or near term, but includes all other sensory systems.

Sensory systems at that stage of development are designed and ready for particular types and amounts of exogenous stimulation. The infant in utero is protected from pain, light, high-frequency sound, and unusual positions or movements. Such stimulation is not required for early development; however, the fetus in utero is exposed to low-frequency sound. Thus, the fetus can hear and develop neural systems in response to speech and music, as well as other low-frequency sounds, such as noise. The auditory system is ready to learn meaningful sounds (language and music) by 31 to 32 weeks' gestation. For the preterm infant in the NICU, it is essential that background neurosensory stimulation (sensory noise) be kept at a level such that sensory systems can discriminate and accommodate meaningful signals or stimulation. This observation is especially true for sound, touch, smell, position, and comfort, which are part of early neurosensory development and in utero learning (or NICU learning).

Learning and memory

Beginning at 28 to 32 weeks' gestational age, sleep and sleep cycles play a critical role in the development of long-term or permanent neurocircuits, and are essential for learning and memory for the life time of an individual. Sleep cycles are an important issue for the infant in the NICU, as well as in the period following NICU discharge [23].

The sequence or process of learning and memory formation consists of three phases as illustrated in Fig. 3 [24]. The first phase in the development of long-term memories (neurocircuits) is the acquisition phase, which occurs during wakefulness. In this phase, the sensory input goes to the neocortex and other areas of the brain where sensory information is stored. Sensory input includes visual, auditory, somatesthetic, olfactory, position, motion, and emotional content. Initially, sensory input is stored in short-term neurocircuits, or memory patterns, which are located in various parts of the neocortex and other brain "storage" areas. Patterns and circuits are not well organized or prioritized for importance or meaning, especially in young infants and toddlers. Inputs from any single sensory system (eg, vision) and its storage are not limited to the visual cortex but are found in many parts of the cortex.

The second phase, learning and memory, is the consolidation phase. When the infant or child goes from wakefulness to sleep, they pass through stage 1 (drowsy or presleep) and stage 2 to stages 3 and 4, NREM slow-wave sleep. During stages 3 or 4 NREM or slow-wave sleep, important short-term memory circuits that are created by sensory input during wakefulness and stored in various parts of the cortex are moved to the hippocampus, para-hippocampal areas, and the amygdala/limbic lobe areas of the temporal lobe. Weak and unimportant signals and stimuli (sensory noise) are eliminated, and important, strong, or salient images and signals are collected in the hippocampal and limbic areas. Signals and images from different sensory systems are integrated and related (see Fig. 3).

The third phase of learning and memory is a period of REM sleep. During REM sleep, there is further organization and integration of short-term memory circuits that were created during wakefulness and consolidated during slow-wave sleep. The P wave from the pons stimulates a process of organization and integration of sensory material in the amygdala, hippocampus, and parahippocampal areas. The generated P wave stimulates the activation of hippocampal theta waves. These theta waves or oscillations create communication between the hippocampus and the neocortex [25]. Through the oscillations of theta waves, neurosensory memory content is returned to the neocortical storage areas, but in an organized and integrated manner; it becomes long-term organized memory circuits that are located in appropriate areas of the brain where they can be recalled or used to build more complex memory patterns [21,22]. This is the learning process. These processes apply to the auditory, touch, position, olfactory, and comfort/emotion systems in preterm infants after 30 to 32 weeks' gestation.

As the infant matures, there are longer awake and sleep periods with several REM-NREM cycles. Sensory input or learning becomes divided, with certain material consolidated and integrated in the first or early NREM-REM cycle and other material and processes consolidated and integrated during the second or third NREM-REM cycles. For children and adults with large amounts of sensory input, stimulation, and learning during a busy day, several cycles of NREM-REM sleep are used to organize and integrate the day's learning into long-term memory circuits. With infants and very young children, the process operates with shorter sleep cycles interspersed with shorter periods of wakefulness.

Preservation of brain plasticity

"Brain plasticity refers to the ability of the brain to persistently change its structure and function according to genetic code in response to environmental changes" [26]. Brain plasticity is an issue for infancy and periods of early brain development, and is critical throughout childhood and adult life. Preservation of brain plasticity is an essential process for the life of an individual.

Sleep deprivation—REM and NREM—in a wide range of animals during brain development resulted in subsequent loss of brain plasticity. This change was manifested by smaller brains, altered subsequent learning, and long-term effects on behavior and brain function [23]. The same effects can be achieved by injury to the hippocampus, pons, or their connections.

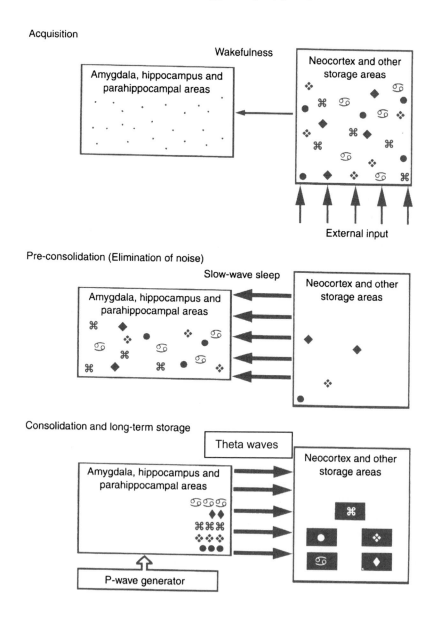

During the early phases of neurosensory development, interference with REM sleep results in loss of normal architecture of sensory nuclei and failure to develop topographic alignment of vision or touch systems. It also interferes with tonographic organization of the auditory system. When these events occur during the critical period of neurosensory development (age 28 weeks' gestation to 3 years of age), there is permanent injury to certain functions as well as loss of future brain plasticity.

There are well-described molecular explanations for the impact of REM sleep deprivation or interference with hippocampal and pons waves on subsequent brain plasticity [27,28]. Facilitation and protection of sleep and sleep cycles are essential to long-term learning and continuing brain development through the preservation of brain plasticity [23,27,28].

Critical components of the sleep cycle that are essential for building the early neurosensory systems, for learning and memory, and for preservation of brain plasticity are shown in Box 1.

These principles and components apply to infants, children, and adults through their lifetime.

Sleep and continuous brain monitoring

Continuous EEG monitoring has provided new technology for following healthy brain activity, as well as the course of brain activity that is associated with injury and insults from a variety of sources. Background electrical activity of the brain evolves rapidly with maturation of the brain beyond 24 weeks' gestational age. Knowledge of this developmental pattern is particularly useful in the NICU. These changes have been recorded with conventional EEG and continuous EEG [5]. The correlation of EEG or continuous EEG patterns with sleep state relies heavily on associated behaviors, including REMs, postural muscle hypotonia, asymmetric cortical

Fig. 3. Model of sleep-dependent memory consolidation and long-term storage. During wakefulness, external information is input randomly into the brain and stored in the neocortex and other storage areas. This process is called acquisition of information. At the time of acquisition, a representational catalog of temporarily stored information is created in the amygdala, hippocampus, and parahippocampal areas. This is an important preconsolidation phase. During this phase, some of the redundant information is eliminated to attenuate signal-to-noise ratio. During the P-wave–related sleep states (tS-R and REM sleep), activation of P-wave–generating cells in the pons reactivates the amygdala, hippocampus and parahippocampal areas to organize the random information acquired during wakefulness. This process is called consolidation of information. Once information is consolidated, it is ready to be stored in the permanent storage. Theta-frequency waves that are generated during REM sleep help to bind that consolidated information into the long-term memory storage in the neocortex and other storage areas. Symbols: five different types of external information. (*Modified from* Datta S. PGO wave generation: mechanisms and functional significance. In: Mallick BN, Inoue S, editors. Rapid eye movement sleep. New Delhi (India): Narosa Publishing House Pvt. Ltd.; 1999. p. 91–106; with permission.)

Box 1. Critical components of the sleep cycle

Wakefulness
Meaningful, appropriate sensory experience
Supportive emotional environment
Absence of conflicting stimuli or excess sensory noise

Non-REM sleep
Cortical slow-wave activity
Hippocampus–cortical oscillations–waves
Sensory system decreased activation
Uninterrupted sleep periods

REM sleep
Desynchronous cortical waves
REMs
Pons-generated P waves and PGO waves
Hippocampus theta waves
Postural muscle atonia (at 2–3 months of age)
Ganglion cell waves (late fetal and early neonatal
   period)–neurosensory development
Uninterrupted sleep periods

---

waves, discontinuous motor activity, and physiologic parameters of heart and respiratory rate and pattern.

Continuous EEG monitoring has not been used for monitoring REM or NREM sleep specifically, although it is observed on many recordings [26,27]. Sleep cycles and patterns that are associated with REM and NREM sleep are seen and reported in the literature on continuous EEG monitoring [5,27]. What is needed is the ability to determine the timing of stage 3 or 4 slow-wave (quiet) sleep with the presence of waves from the hippocampus and parahippocampus area. If these waves are suppressed, there will be little consolidation of the sensory input to build neurosensory systems or to support learning and long-term memory. Also needed is the ability to determine the presence and status of the P wave or PGO waves that are generated in the pons and theta waves that are generated by the hippocampus, which are associated with endogenous waves that are required for building neurosensory systems as well as continued learning, memory, and preservation of brain plasticity.

With the increasing use of midazolam and other medications to suppress seizures, quiet infants, or treat cardiac, pulmonary, or gastrointestinal problems, the effect of medications on critical elements of REM and NREM sleep and sleep cycles becomes important in the protection of brain development and improving long-term outcome.

Thus, continuous sleep monitoring, and especially the ability to monitor critical EEG/brain wave elements of the REM/NREM sleep cycle, will be an important and much-needed advance in the technology of continuous brain monitoring. Only with the ability to monitor sleep and its EEG components will it be possible to study the impact of NICU medication, events, and environment on the processes of early brain development. This step is essential for understanding the factors that are responsible for the many and varied neurologic, behavioral, and learning issues that are found in long-term follow-up of preterm infants.

Further readings

Hobson JA. Sleep. New York: Scientific American Library; 1995.

Iversen S, Kupfermann I, Kandel ER. Emotional states and feelings. In: Kandel ER, Schwartz JH, Jessell TM, editors. Principles of neural science. New York: McGraw-Hill; 2000. p. 982–97.

Lagercratz H, Hanson M, Evrard P, et al. The newborn brain: neuroscience and clinical application. New York: Cambridge University Press; 2002.

Mallick BN, Inoue S. Rapid eye movement sleep. New York: Marcel Dekker; 1999.

Marquet P, Smith C, Stickgold R. Sleep and brain plasticity. New York: Oxford University Press; 2003.

Rechtschaffen A, Siegel J. Sleep and dreaming. In: Kandel ER, Schwartz JH, Jessell TM, editors. Principles of neural science. New York: McGraw-Hill; 2000. p. 936–47.

Turek F, Lee P. Regulation of sleep and circadian rhythms. New York: Marcel Dekker; 1999.

References

[1] Loomis AL, Harvey EN, Hobart GA. Electrical potentials of the human brain. J Exp Psychol 1936;19:249–79.

[2] Aserinsky E, Kleitman N. Regularly occurring periods of eye motility and concomitant phenomena, during sleep. Science 1953;118:273–4.

[3] Dement NC, Kleitman N. Cyclic variations in EEG during sleep and their relation to eye movements, body motility and dreaming. Electroencephalogr Clin Neurophysiol 1957;9: 673–90.

[4] Rechtschaffen A, Kales A, editors. A manual of standardized terminology, techniques, and scoring system for sleep stages of human subjects. Los Angeles (CA): UCLA Brain Information Service/Brain Research Institute; 1968.

[5] Stickgold R. Human studies of sleep and off-line memory reprocessing. In: Maquet P, Smith C, Stickgold R, editors. Sleep and brain plasticity. New York: Oxford University Press; 2003. p. 41–64.

[6] Nader R, Smith C. A role for stage 2 sleep in memory processing. In: Maquet P, Smith C, Stickgold R, editors. Sleep and brain plasticity. New York: Oxford University Press; 2003. p. 87–98.

[7] Hobson JA. The neurology of sleep. In: Sleep. New York: Scientific American Library; 1995. p. 118–41.

[8] Lai Y-Y, Siegel JM. Muscle atonia in REM sleep. In: Mallick BN, Inouí S, editors. Rapid eye movement sleep. New Delhi (India): Narosa Publishing House Pvt. Ltd; 1999. p. 69–90.

[9] Davis FC, Frank MG, Heller HC. Ontogeny of sleep and circadian rhythms. In: Turek FW, Zee PC, editors. Regulation of sleep and circadian rhythms. New York: Marcel Dekker; 1999. p. 19–79.

[10] Hobson J. The development of sleep. In: Sleep. New York: Scientific American Library; 1995. p. 71–91.

[11] Segawa M. Ontogenesis of REM sleep. In: Mallick B, Inouí S, editors. Rapid eye movement sleep. New Delhi (India): Narosa Publishing House Pvt. Ltd; 1999. p. 9–50.

[12] Mizrahi EM, Hrachovy RA, Kellaway P. Atlas of neonatal electroencephalography. Philadelphia: Lippincott Williams and Wilkins; 2004.

[13] Hellstrom-Westas L, de Vries L, Rosen I. An atlas of amplitude- integrated EEG's in the newborn. Boca Raton (FL): Parthenon Publishing Group; 2003.

[14] Clancy RR, Chung HJ, Temple JP. Atlas of electroencephalography. Amsterdam: Elsevier; 1999.

[15] Dreyfus-Brisac C. Neurophysiological studies in human premature and full-term newborns. Biol Psychiatry 1975;10(5):485–96.

[16] Datta S. Avoidance task training potentiates phasic pontine-wave density in the rat: a mechanism for sleep-dependent plasticity. J Neurosci 2000;20:8607–13.

[17] Okai T, Kozuma S, Shinozuka N, et al. A study on the development of sleep-wakefulness cycle in the human fetus. Early Hum Dev 1992;29(1–3):391–6.

[18] Penn AA, Shatz CJ. Principles of endogenous and sensory activity dependent brain development. The visual system. In: Lagercrantz H, Hanson M, Evrard P, editors. The newborn brain: neuroscience and clinical applications. New York: Cambridge University Press; 2002. p. 204–25.

[19] Penn AA, Shatz CJ. Brain waves and brain wiring: the role of endogenous and sensory-driven neural activity in development. Pediatr Res 1999;45(4 Pt 1):447–58.

[20] Graven SN. Early neurosensory visual development of the fetus and newborn. Clin Perinatol 2004;31(2):199–216.

[21] Palmer SE. Vision science: photons to phenomenology. Cambridge (MA): MIT Press; 1999.

[22] Frank MG, Stryker MP. The role of sleep in the development of central visual pathways. In: Maquet P, Smith C, Stickgold R, editors. Sleep and brain plasticity. New York: Oxford University Press; 2003. p. 87–98.

[23] Maquet P, Smith C, Stickgold R. Sleep and brain plasticity. New York: Oxford University Press; 2003.

[24] Datta S. PGO wave generation: mechanisms and functional significance. In: Mallick BN, Inoue S, editors. Rapid eye movement sleep. New Delhi (India): Narosa Publishing House Pvt. Ltd; 1999. p. 91–106.

[25] Datta S, Patterson EH. Activation of phasic pontine wave (P-wave): a mechanism of learning and memory processing. In: Maquet P, Smith C, Stickgold R, editors. Sleep and brain plasticity. New York: Oxford University Press; 2003. p. 135–56.

[26] Maquet P, Smith C, Stickgold R. Introduction. In: Maquet P, Smith C, Stickgold R, editors. Sleep and brain plasticity. New York: Oxford University Press; 2003. p. 1–13.

[27] Mirmiran M, Ariagno RL. Role of REM sleep in brain development and plasticity. In: Maquet P, Smith C, Stickgold R, editors. Sleep and brain plasticity. New York: Oxford University Press; 2003. p. 181–7.

[28] Nedivi E. Molecular analysis of developmental plasticity in neocortex. J Neurobiol 1999; 41(1):135–47.

ELSEVIER
SAUNDERS

Clin Perinatol 33 (2006) 707–728

CLINICS IN
PERINATOLOGY

Near-Infrared Spectroscopy in the Fetus and Neonate

Adam J. Wolfberg, MD, MPH[a,b,c],
Adré J. du Plessis, MBChB, MPH[a,b,*]

[a]*Department of Neurology, Children's Hospital Boston,
300 Longwood Avenue, Boston, MA 02115, USA*
[b]*Department of Neurology, Harvard Medical School, 25 Shattuck Street Boston,
MA 02115, USA*
[c]*Department of Obstetrics and Gynecology, Tufts New England Medical Center,
Washington Street, Boston, MA 02115, USA*

Near-infrared spectroscopy (NIRS) was introduced in 1977 as a technology that is capable of noninvasive monitoring of oxygenation in living tissue [1]. NIRS operates on the principle that near-infrared (NIR) light (700–1000 nm) passes easily through tissue and is absorbed in an oxygen-dependent manner by chromophores that include hemoglobin and cytochrome aa_3 [1]. The use of NIRS to study changes in oxygenation and hemodynamics in the brain of the human newborn was described first by Brazy and colleagues in 1985 [2]. Although portable NIRS devices are small enough to be used in the close quarters of the neonatal ICU or in the operating room, and have been used as a research tool by neurologists, neonatologists, cardiac surgeons, and anesthesiologists to study cerebral hemodynamics and oxygenation, the technology has yet to gain widespread acceptance as a technology for routine clinical monitoring [3].

Principles of near-infrared spectroscopy

Light in the NIR range (the portion of the infrared range closest to the visual spectrum, or 700–1000 nm) easily penetrates soft tissue and bone, particularly the thin tissues and skull of the neonate. Chromophores—chemical groups that are capable of NIR light absorption, including circulating hemoglobin, as well as tissue cytochrome aa_3 and myoglobin—absorb this

---

* Corresponding author. Department of Neurology, Children's Hospital Boston, 300 Longwood Avenue, Boston, MA 02115.
E-mail address: adre.duplessis@childrens.harvard.edu (A.J. du Plessis).

0095-5108/06/$ - see front matter © 2006 Elsevier Inc. All rights reserved.
doi:10.1016/j.clp.2006.06.010 *perinatology.theclinics.com*

transmitted light at quantifiably different amounts depending on their oxygenation state. NIRS devices use NIR light at wavelengths that correspond to the wavelengths of maximal absorption for the relevant chromophores. NIRS measures changes in tissue concentration of oxyhemoglobin and deoxyhemoglobin, and from the summation of these measurements derives changes in total cerebral hemoglobin concentrations.

NIRS also measures changes in the concentration of oxidized intracellular cytochrome aa_3, the terminal enzyme in the mitochondrial electron transport chain, and the final electron donor to molecular oxygen. Changes in the concentration of oxidized cytochrome aa_3 reflect the availability of oxygen to the mitochondria, the delivery of reducing substances to the electron transport chain, and the rate of ATP turnover [4]. Information on cytochrome aa_3 is useful because it provides a measure of intracellular oxygenation.

A modification of the Beer-Lambert law ($A = \alpha BdC + G$) describes the relationship between the absorption of NIR light and the absorbing chromophore's concentration in tissue, where A is the attenuation measured in units of optical density, α is the specific absorption coefficient of the chromophore at a particular wavelength ($\mu molar^{-1} \cdot cm^{-1}$), B is the differential pathlength factor (DPF), d is the distance between NIRS optodes (cm), C is the concentration of the chromophore in the tissue ($\mu mol/L$), and G is an additive term that represents the scattering losses of NIR light as it passes through the tissue. All coefficients in the equation, except for the DPF, are known constants or can be measured. The DPF is known for several different biologic tissues, although variation in the DPF between subjects may explain, in part, why standardization of NIRS parameters across subjects has been difficult [5].

Types of near-infrared spectroscopy devices

Continuous wave near-infrared spectroscopy devices

The most frequently used NIRS device for human and animal studies is the continuous wave spectrometer, which uses lasers to generate NIR light at different wavelengths. Light is transmitted by way of fiber-optic cables into the brain, where photons scatter and are absorbed. The remaining light is transmitted back to the device, and the absorbance at selected wavelengths is converted into a change in concentration of the relevant chromophore using an algorithm that is specific to the wavelength of light.

One problem with this technique, in which the precise pathlength of NIR light is unknown, is that it only measures absolute change in the concentration of chromophores and requires biochemical or hemodynamic changes to occur in tissues for these measurements to be made. Systems that are designed to measure the absolute value of oxygen saturation levels have demonstrated considerable variability when compared with alternative monitoring systems, as well as significant interpatient variability [6,7].

Time-resolved near-infrared spectroscopy devices

The time-resolved NIRS devices measure the time that is required for a picosecond pulse of light to pass through tissue. These systems have the advantage of measuring the actual pathlength of light, and from an analysis of the returning light are able to measure absolute concentrations of chromophores [8]. Technical requirements of this technology have made it extremely expensive, and it requires more space than typically is available at the bedside of a neonate.

Phase-resolved spectroscopy

Phase-resolved spectroscopy measures the amplitude and phase shift of light that can be calculated when light of a certain frequency is used. These variables are modulated by the tissue that the light has passed through, which can be accounted for in a calculation that allows for the quantification of oxygen saturation. In theory, this technique allows for the measurement of the absolute concentration of oxyhemoglobin and deoxyhemoglobin, and, hence, total hemoglobin and cerebral blood volume. These calculations are based on assumptions about the homogeneity of measured tissue, however, which may affect the accuracy of measurements [8].

Using near-infrared spectroscopy to measure cerebral hemodynamic and oxygenation variables of interest

NIRS can measure the absolute changes in oxyhemoglobin and deoxyhemoglobin concentrations directly, and, with some straightforward calculations, can be used to derive additional hemodynamic variables of clinical interest. Validation of NIRS measurements has proved challenging because there are few alternative methods for measuring changes in cerebral oxygenation that can serve as a gold standard. One study that compared NIRS with peripheral pulse oximetry found strong correlation between the two technologies for large changes in oxygenation, but poor correlation for smaller changes [9]. Changes in oxyhemoglobin and deoxyhemoglobin may be measured continuously and compared with measurements of systemic variables, including oxygen saturation, heart rate, and blood pressure, which provide the researcher with an indication of the cerebral hemodynamic response to systemic hemodynamic events.

NIRS also may be used to calculate point measurements of cerebral hemodynamic status. Absolute cerebral blood volume can be calculated using the indicator-dilution technique during the induction of 5% to 10% changes in circulating oxyhemoglobin saturation (within the range of 80%–95%) over several minutes by changing inspired oxygen concentrations. Absolute cerebral blood volume is calculated by plotting the change in cerebral oxyhemoglobin (NIRS) against the change in systemic oxyhemoglobin concentration (pulse oximetry) using the formula:

$$\text{Cerebral blood volume} = (\Delta[\text{HbO}_2] - \Delta[\text{Hb}])/(2 \cdot \text{SaO}_2 \cdot H \cdot R)$$

where HbO_2 is oxyhemoglobin, Hb is deoxyhemoglobin, SaO_2 is arterial oxygen saturation, H is the large vessel hemoglobin concentration, and R is the cerebral-to-large vessel hematocrit ratio [10,11]. NIRS measurement of cerebral blood volume has been validated against strain gauge plethysmography, with good correlation between the two techniques [12].

Cerebral blood flow also can be calculated using inspired oxygen as a "marker" and applying the Fick principle, which states that the amount of substance consumed by an organ can be calculated by subtracting the rate of the substance's departure from the rate of the substance's arrival at the organ [13]. Using this "oxygen bolus" technique, measurements are made over a period less than the "known" cerebral transit time of hemoglobin. Therefore, it is assumed that over this brief time period all changes in oxyhemoglobin concentration measured by NIRS are due to accumulation only. By comparing the curves of the changing systemic oxyhemoglobin saturation (pulse oximetry) and the changing cerebral oxyhemoglobin concentration during this brief period, cerebral blood flow can be derived by the formula:

$$\text{Cerebral blood flow} = K_1 \cdot \Delta[\text{HbO}_2/\text{HbT}] \cdot f_0^t(\Delta(\text{SaO}_2)dt)$$

where K_1 is a constant reflecting the molecular weight of hemoglobin (64,500), HbO_2 is oxyhemoglobin, HbT is total hemoglobin, and SaO_2 is arterial oxygen saturation [13–16]. NIRS measurement of cerebral blood flow has been compared with measurement of the cerebral blood flow by [133]Xenon clearance, an established method, with good correlation [15]. Cerebral blood flow also can be measured by using a bolus of indocyanine green, a dye that is injected into peripheral circulation and is cleared rapidly by the liver. Because indocyanine green has peak NIR light absorption around the same wavelength of cytochrome aa3, the NIRS cytochrome aa3 curve following a bolus of the indocyanine green tracer can be used to calculate cerebral blood flow. If indocyanine green is used, its concentration change in systemic circulation must be measured by using a separate device [14]. More recently, noninvasive methods for measurement of systemic indocyanine green concentration changes have been described [17,18].

Cerebral venous oxygen saturation has been calculated by measuring the change in hemoglobin concentrations during procedures that cause a brief change in cerebral venous volume. Such techniques include a sudden head tilt or brief jugular occlusion, the assumption being that the resulting brief cerebral blood volume changes are confined to the cerebral venous compartment. The oxyhemoglobin saturation of cerebral venous blood is derived using the formula:

$$\text{Cerebral venous saturation} = \Delta[HbO_2]/\Delta[HbT]$$

where HbO_2 is oxyhemoglobin and HbT is total hemoglobin, which is the sum of oxyhemoglobin and deoxyhemoglobin. This method has been validated with blood sampled from the jugular bulb during cardiac catheterization [19,20].

Cerebral carbon dioxide vasoreactivity can be assessed by measuring the cerebral hemodynamic response to changes in the circulating Pco_2, induced by modest changes in the ventilator rate. Wyatt and colleagues [21] found a linear increase in cerebral blood volume in response to increasing CO_2 levels, and although Brun and Greisen [22] found the same trend, there was poor consistency between CO_2 vasoreactivity responses that were elicited by changing ventilator settings to affect levels and the responses that were generated by using the oxygen tracer method. The various cerebral hemodynamic parameters measured by the above techniques have been applied to derive other valuable measures, including cerebral oxygen metabolism, cerebral oxygen delivery and fractional oxygen extraction (the ratio between oxygen metabolism and oxygen delivery), and total circulating blood volume [23–25]. One potential limitation of the "static" hemodynamic measurements that were described above is the assumption that other variables (eg, oxygen metabolism, cerebral blood volume, cerebral blood flow) remain constant and do not interact during the period of measurement, an assumption that is not well established by using alternative methods of quantification [3,24]. One study that used NIRS during cardiac catheterization to calculate the percent contribution to cerebral oxygenation measurements of arterial and venous blood found significant variation between subjects in this measurement [26]; this suggested that the hemodynamic parameters that are assumed to be constant may be anything but.

Specific clinical applications of near-infrared spectroscopy

Studies in the fetus

The holy grail of fetal monitoring is a reliable, accurate way of measuring fetal cerebral oxygenation levels. Despite decades of research, fetal heart rate monitoring, fetal pulse oximetry, and ultrasound testing have not been demonstrated to meet this challenge with sufficient sensitivity to reduce fetal or neonatal hypoxic-ischemic injury. Several investigators have explored the ability of NIRS to provide a measure of fetal cerebral oxygenation during the antepartum and even intrapartum periods.

Antepartum fetal NIRS is complicated by the technical challenge of collecting data through the maternal abdomen, which not only presents the challenge of localization—knowing that the optodes are measuring light refracted through fetal tissue—but also of incorporating refraction from maternal tissue in the analysis of the recorded data. One study of late-term pregnant women placed the optodes of the NIRS device on the maternal abdomen in a location measured in relation to the fetal head as identified by ultrasound [27]. The intraoptode distance was set to be twice the depth of the fetal head from the abdominal surface. Fetal cerebral oxygen saturation measured in this manner ranged from 50% to 74%; however, there is currently no way to validate these data. Using a similar configuration, another group measured placental oxygenation, although with similar limitations [28].

NIRS has been used in fetal animal studies to elucidate changes in cerebral oxygenation during intrauterine asphyxia. Bennet and colleagues [29] studied instrumented premature fetal sheep for 3 days following 30 minutes of cord occlusion, and found that 3 to 5 hours after occlusion there was a significant reduction in cerebral blood flow, blood volume, and oxygenation, despite normal perfusion pressure and heart rate. In a more recent study, this group found that cerebral oxygenation decreased transiently 3 to 4 hours after cord occlusion, but then increased dramatically to greater than control levels thereafter [30]. Cytochrome aa_3 oxidation levels decreased significantly, which indicated a loss in mitochondrial activity and secondary energy failure hours after asphyxia. Newman and colleagues [31] tested the effect of an adenosine bolus on the fetus' ability to tolerate hypoxia, and found that cerebral oxygenation increased, whereas cerebral cytochrome aa_3 became more oxidized, which suggested a decrease in metabolic rate. Peebles and colleagues [32] used NIRS to evaluate cerebral oxygenation in premature fetal sheep after injection of *Escherichia coli* lipopolysaccharide. They found a decrease in oxyhemoglobin and an increase in deoxyhemoglobin after lipopolysaccharide administration in the context of a significant increase in cerebral blood flow and a decrease in systemic blood pressure, presumably in response to the *E coli* endotoxin. They concluded that hypoxia is not the mediating factor in the development of white matter injury in neonates who are exposed to intrauterine infection. These studies in animal models demonstrate the potential usefulness of NIRS for evaluating cerebral oxygenation during invasive experiments that model conditions of fetal asphyxia.

Intrapartum NIRS measurements of human fetuses have been made by transvaginal placement of the optodes directly on the fetal head after rupture of membranes and sufficient cervical dilation. The first studies that used NIRS during labor reported a decline in fetal cerebral oxyhemoglobin, deoxyhemoglobin, and total hemoglobin during maternal contractions, and calculated a decrease in cerebral blood volume that was due to compression of the fetal head [33,34]. In Peebles and colleagues' [33] study, however, when fetal heart rate decelerations occurred during contractions, total hemoglobin and oxyhemoglobin decreased, and deoxyhemoglobin increased, which suggested cerebral oxygen desaturation. In other studies, this pattern was more pronounced during contractions that were accompanied by late fetal heart rate decelerations than during contractions that were not accompanied by fetal heart rate decelerations [35,36]. The interval between contractions also was associated with the change in cerebral oxyhemoglobin, and inversely with the change in deoxyhemoglobin [35]. In another study, similar changes were noted in a nonviable fetus, however [37]. In these studies, the hemoglobin signals returned to baseline after contractions, and none of the monitored neonates were born with clinically significant acidemia or depression as measured by Apgar scores. These studies did, however, demonstrate that trends measured using NIRS were associated with trends measured using fetal heat rate and contraction monitors in a temporal manner that made physiologic sense.

Peebles and colleagues calculated fetal cerebral oxygenation using changes in the concentration of oxyhemoglobin and deoxyhemoglobin and demonstrated a strong correlation between their measurement of cerebral oxygenation just before delivery and umbilical artery and umbilical vein pH measured immediately after delivery in a study of 33 fetuses who had an umbilical arterial pH range of 7.09 to 7.43 [38] This is an important study, because it uses cord blood measures of fetal oxygenation to validate the technique, a superior measure to fetal heart rate changes, which are only weakly predictive of fetal distress. There are, however, significant concerns about these calculated fetal cerebral oxygenation NIRS measurements. First, these measurements require that oxyhemoglobin and deoxyhemoglobin change in the same direction, an unusual phenomenon during fetal distress. Furthermore, the measurement represents mixed arterial and venous blood, and does not account for oxygen extraction—an important variable that may be altered significantly by preceding cerebral cellular injury.

Other limitations of intrapartum cerebral NIRS recordings include significant movement artifact; up to 30% to 40% of data recorded in early studies could not be analyzed because of the poor quality of the data. Second, correlating baseline NIRS data with pulse oximetry or blood gas measurements—admittedly also a problem in neonates—is particularly difficult when recording data from a fetus. Another study that compared fetal pulse oximetry with fetal NIRS measurements found that systemic oxygen saturation by pulse oximetry was correlated positively with NIRS-measured cerebral oxyhemoglobin and total hemoglobin, and negatively with deoxyhemoglobin concentrations [39]. These and other practical problems with the technology have impeded the implementation of fetal NIRS monitoring to the clinical management of labor.

Studies in preterm and term neonates

Much of the research using NIRS has focused on preterm and term newborns because so many of the neurologic injuries that occur in the population involve ongoing or pre-existing disturbances of cerebral perfusion and oxygen delivery. Furthermore, because the skin and skull of the newborn, particularly the premature newborn, is highly permeable to NIR light, this group of subjects is well suited to research using this technology.

Early studies with this population focused on validating calculated NIRS measurements and establishing normative data [14–16,21]. A common theme in these reports was the wide variation between measurements on the same subject and on different subjects, which compromised the reliability and validity of the technology. Using the oxyhemoglobin indicator dilution technique, mean cerebral blood volume in the term newborn was 2.22 ± 0.40 mL/100 g [11]. Carbon dioxide vasoreactivity also was measured by altering the $Paco_2$ by changing the ventilator respiratory rate. Vasoreactivity to CO_2 increased with gestational age from 0.07 mL/100 g/kPa at 26 weeks' gestational age to 0.51 mL/100 g/kPa of change in CO_2 at term [21]. A study of healthy newborns also found that cerebral CO_2 vasoreactivity increased with postnatal age [40]. Cerebral blood flow was quantified using the oxygen marker method, and ranged from 5 to 30 mL/100 g/min between 25 and 44 weeks [13–16]. Two of these studies validated the NIRS method of measuring cerebral blood flow with the [133]Xenon method and found good correlation between the two techniques ($r = 0.8$ and $r = 0.84$) [15,16]. Patel and colleagues [14] compared the oxygen bolus and indocyanine green methods of measuring cerebral blood flow and demonstrated good correlation between the two techniques in a study of six neonates; however, there was intrasubject variation in cerebral blood flow of between 15% and 40%. Weiss and colleagues [41] evaluated the variance in cerebral oxygenation measured with NIRS. Although variance between measurements could not be explained wholly, venous oxygen saturation and the presence or absence of a cardiac shunt explained a significant amount of the variance.

Studies of apneic events using NIRS demonstrated inconsistent changes in cerebral blood volume [42,43]; however, cerebral blood volume is influenced by several hemodynamic variables, such that the apneic event itself is only one factor. In one study, NIRS recordings of 130 apneic episodes (central, obstructive, or mixed apnea) showed a decrease in cerebral blood volume in most infants; however, 12% of infants showed no change in cerebral blood volume and 28% showed an increase in cerebral blood volume. The study also demonstrated no correlation between the change in cerebral blood volume and the lowest oxygen saturation level recorded, which suggested that apnea alone does not influence cerebral blood volume [44]. Other investigators found cerebral blood volume to decrease during apneas along with cerebral oxygenation [45,46]. Another study of spontaneous apneic episodes in preterm neonates found that although hypoxia was not associated with a change in total hemoglobin concentrations measured by NIRS, apneic spells that were associated with bradycardias did demonstrate a significant decline in total hemoglobin concentrations [47]. These findings suggest that the decrease in cardiac output during a period of bradycardia overwhelmed the capacity of the premature brain to vasodilate when facing hypoxic conditions. This hypothesis is supported by research that showed that although cerebral oxygenation and cerebral blood volume were unaffected in a group of premature neonates that had apnea and normal heart rate, these variables decreased in a group that had apnea and bradycardia, even though peripheral oxygenation decreased in both groups [48]. These findings emphasize the importance of measuring as many potentially relevant physiologic variables as possible when using NIRS in studies of cerebral hemodynamics so that an appropriate model—that includes all relevant physiologic mechanisms—may be constructed.

NIRS has been used to evaluate the effect of medications that are used to treat apnea on cerebral oxygenation. Aminophylline, once used widely, was associated with significant changes in cerebral blood volume and cerebral blood flow [49,50]. Caffeine did not affect these parameters [50]. Doxapram decreased oxyhemoglobin levels, presumably by increasing oxygen consumption [51]. Use of indomethacin was associated with a significant decline in cerebral blood volume, cerebral blood flow, cerebral oxygen delivery, and carbon dioxide vasoreactivity [52–54], whereas ibuprofen was not [55]. Indomethacin use also was associated with a substantial decline in oxidized cytochrome aa_3, which suggested cellular hypoxia as well [53].

Near-infrared spectroscopy as a monitor of cerebral hemodynamics

Because impaired cerebral pressure autoregulation in preterm neonates may contribute to the development of cerebrovascular injuries, such as periventricular leukomalacia and germinal matrix intraventricular hemorrhage [56], particular attention has been focused on the capacity of NIRS to elucidate the process of cerebral pressure autoregulation in preterm infants. Tyszczuk and colleagues [57] made static cerebral blood flow measurements using the oxygen bolus technique every 2 to 3 hours in one group of preterm neonates with mean arterial blood pressure greater than 30 mm Hg. They compared these with another group with mean arterial blood pressure of less than 30 mm Hg. There was no correlation between the mean arterial blood pressure and the mean cerebral blood flow in individual infants, and no difference in cerebral blood flow between groups. Although the investigators concluded that these subjects had intact cerebral autoregulation, the study was not designed to capture dynamic changes in cerebral blood flow, mean arterial pressure, and the interrelationship between the variables, because cerebral blood flow was measured only intermittently during 2- to 3-hour study periods, so the dynamic relationship between variables could not be established.

Dynamic monitoring of cerebral pressure and autoregulation

Other investigators have evaluated instantaneous changes in hemodynamic variables to construct a correlation model that is more dynamic.

The authors' group studied 32 ventilated premature infants ranging in gestational age from 23 weeks to 31 weeks (mean 27 weeks) [58]. All infants had indwelling umbilical arterial catheters for clinically indicated continuous blood pressure monitoring. In a subset of 17 (53%) infants, they described concordant changes in mean arterial pressure and changes in the cerebral "hemoglobin difference." The signal representing hemoglobin difference (oxyhemoglobin minus deoxyhemoglobin) has been validated as a surrogate for cerebral blood flow in animals [59,60]. Of these 17 infants, 8 (47%) developed severe intraventricular hemorrhage (grades III/IV) or periventricular leukomalacia, compared with only 2 (13%) of 15 infants with apparently independent changes in systemic pressure and cerebral hemoglobin (ie, suggesting intact cerebral autoregulation) [58]. Among the 10 studied neonates who had severe ultrasound abnormalities, 8 showed significant concordance between changes in blood pressure and hemoglobin difference [59], which supports the premise that a subset of sick neonates may have pressure-passive circulation and are at higher risk for subsequent neurologic injury.

Sick neonates have been evaluated using NIRS to identify risk factors for a loss of cerebral autoregulation. Munro and colleagues [61] correlated cerebral blood flow with mean arterial pressure in a group of hypotensive and normotensive premature neonates, and collected NIRS data during management of hypotension with dopamine. They found a correlation between mean arterial pressure and cerebral blood flow only when mean arterial pressure was less than 30 mm Hg, which suggested that autoregulation was present in normotensive neonates. Similarly, Pellicer and colleagues [62] found a correlation between mean arterial pressure and cerebral oxygenation in hypotensive neonates who were receiving inotropic agents to increase pressure.

Another line of NIRS investigation that has shed light on cerebral pressure autoregulation came from a study that used NIRS to measure fractional oxygen extraction in a group of preterm neonates [25]. In this study, oxygen extraction was similar in neonates who had hypotension, moderate anemia, and changing Pco_2 levels. This led the investigators to hypothesize that an intact system of cerebral autoregulation maintained perfusion in these neonates, which compensated for conditions that might otherwise affect oxygen delivery (eg, hypotension, anemia). Kissack and colleagues [20] also noted in a study of extremely premature neonates that oxygen extraction is related inversely to cerebral blood flow.

Lemmers and colleagues [63] used NIRS to study preterm infants who had respiratory distress syndrome (RDS). Although overall cerebral oxygenation and oxygen extraction did not differ between infants who had RDS and control infants, there was more variance in these variables among neonates who had RDS. Furthermore, infants who had RDS demonstrated more periods of correlation between systemic blood pressure and NIRS measures of cerebral oxygenation and oxygen extraction. This suggested that infants with higher overall illness severity scores are more likely to develop impaired cerebral pressure autoregulation.

Cerebral hemodynamics during interventions in the neonatal ICU

The relationships between cerebral hemodynamics and procedures that are performed during care of the sick preterm neonate have been studied by NIRS. The use of NIRS during the removal of cerebral spinal fluid in cases of posthemorrhagic hydrocephalus demonstrated significant increases in cerebral blood volume, oxyhemoglobin, and oxidized cytochrome aa_3 [64–66]. Slow sampling of blood from a umbilical artery catheter avoided a decrease in cerebral oxygenation measured with NIRS that was caused by fast blood sampling in one study [67]; however, another report found that the decrease in oxygenation could not be prevented by slow sampling [68]. Not unexpectedly, a study of neonates who underwent blood-product transfusions found that cerebral oxyhemoglobin and deoxyhemoglobin increased after transfusion, whereas cerebral blood volume decreased, presumably as a result of increased vascular tone [51]. Gavage feedings reduced cerebral blood volume and oxyhemoglobin concentrations in premature neonates [69]. The mechanism for this response is not clear but presumably involves changes in autonomic tone.

NIRS has been used to evaluate cerebral hemodynamics during mechanical ventilation and during suctioning in ventilated newborns, albeit with conflicting results. Intermittent positive pressure ventilation and continuous negative extrathoracic pressure ventilation are associated with reduced cerebral blood flow, albeit by small amounts [70]. Shah and colleagues [42] found that endotracheal suctioning was associated with a decrease in peripheral and cerebral hemoglobin saturation and an increase in cerebral blood volume in 12 preterm infants who were studied using NIRS. They also found that these changes could be prevented by oxygenating the newborn before suctioning. Another report found that suctioning was not associated with a significant decrease in cerebral blood volume, and that there was no significant difference in cerebral or peripheral oxygen saturation between open and closed suctioning [43]. The type of ventilator—conventional or high-frequency oscillatory—did not affect oxygenation during suctioning [71]. NIRS studies in infants who had congenital heart disease showed that a hypercapnic-inspired gas mixture increased cerebral oxygenation and mean arterial blood pressure in neonates with single-ventricle physiology, whereas a hypoxic gas mixture had no effect on these parameters [72]. Other studies showed that ventilation with hypoxic gas may improve cerebral oxygenation in infants who have congenital heart disease that is associated with increased pulmonary blood flow [73].

Investigations that evaluated the cerebral response that is associated with surfactant administration have reported inconsistent results, with studies

demonstrating an increase [74], mixed results [75], or no change [76] in cerebral blood volume.

Asphyxiated neonates have been the subject of several studies that evaluated the use of NIRS to measure cerebral hemodynamics in the first hours
of life in an effort to elucidate the patterns and time-course of injury. As
therapies for the treatment of asphyxiated newborns emerge, NIRS has
the potential to be useful in studies that evaluate the effect of these therapies
and interventions. A study of severely asphyxiated term newborns found significant decreases in cerebral blood volume, oxyhemoglobin, and cytochrome aa_3 compared with normal control infants or infants who had
moderate asphyxia and did not have neurologic abnormalities at follow-up
[77]. Meek and colleagues [78] showed that perinatal asphyxia was associated with an increase in cerebral blood flow and cerebral blood volume during the first 24 hours of life, as well as a significant reduction in cerebral
carbon dioxide vasoreactivity. Other investigators also reported that severely asphyxiated newborns who were treated with high-dose allopurinol
had a smaller decrease in cerebral blood volume compared with untreated
controls [79]. Toet and colleagues [80] also demonstrated an increase in
regional cerebral oxygen saturation using NIRS and a decline in oxygen
extraction among asphyxiated neonates who died compared with
asphyxiated neonates with a normal long-term outcome. As a predictor of
long-term outcome, measured at up to 5 years of age, abnormal amplitude-
integrated EEG values at 24 hours of life were more predictive of outcome
than were NIRS data in this study.

Investigators have used NIRS to evaluate the cerebral oxygenation and
hemodynamics of term and preterm neonates who were subjected to
a wide variety of pathologic conditions and interventions. An increased
awareness of cerebral autoregulation and the subtle effects that routine interventions can have on cerebral hemodynamics are among the most significant contributions of this technology. Despite these contributions, the
inability of NIRS to measure absolute concentrations and the poor reliability of measurements have worked to keep NIRS largely within the research
domain in the neonatal ICU.

Evaluating infants during or following cardiac surgery

Changes in cerebral hemodynamics and oxygenation during cardiopulmonary bypass and deep hypothermic circulatory arrest are complex and
may have profound effects on the infant's neurologic status in the short
and long term. Because the hemodynamic conditions are changing rapidly, the capacity of NIRS to provide continuous real-time information
about changes in cerebral hemodynamics and oxygenation status that likely
underlie the development of brain injury in this setting triggered a growing
body of intraoperative data generated by NIRS. Early studies during

cardiopulmonary bypass showed an initial decrease in total hemoglobin, presumably due to hemodilution used during cardiopulmonary bypass [81,82]. During this decrease in total hemoglobin, there was an increase in oxyhemoglobin and a decrease in deoxyhemoglobin, which suggested decreased cerebral oxygen extraction during cooling [81–84]. Kurth and colleagues [83] showed in a study of 26 children who underwent cardiac surgery with deep hypothermic circulatory arrest that 3 children who developed postoperative neurologic abnormalities had a smaller increase in cerebral hemoglobin oxygen saturation and a shorter duration of bypass before cooling compared with normal children. Cerebral hemoglobin oxygenation measured by NIRS correlates well with jugular bulb venous saturation [85], an estimate of cerebral oxygen extraction under conditions where arterial blood is saturated fully with oxygen during bypass. Correlation with central venous oxygen saturation also was high, but NIRS measurements varied significantly between patients and between measurements [86].

Research with NIRS has demonstrated that although oxyhemoglobin increases during the cooling phase of these surgeries, oxidized cytochrome aa_3 decreases, which suggests an uncoupling of cerebral intravascular and mitochondrial oxygenation [82,84]. This decrease in cytochrome aa_3 continued throughout bypass and deep hypothermic circulatory arrest and demonstrated delayed recovery during rewarming, despite a recovery of oxyhemoglobin to levels above baseline, presumably as a result of hyperemic reperfusion [82]. That the decline in oxidized cytochrome aa_3 continued after the minimum core temperature was reached suggested that the decrease in oxidized cytochrome aa_3 was not due to hypothermia alone, but that an intrinsic mitochondrial dysfunction or failure of oxygen delivery to the mitochondrion occurred. It is hypothesized that these disturbances underlie a failure in cellular energy metabolism, and, therefore, play a role in the development of brain injury. This study found that these patterns of oxidized cytochrome aa_3 behavior were more pronounced in infants who were older than 14 days, which suggests maturational vulnerability of the mitochondrion to hypoxic-ischemic stress, possibly caused by increased energy demands or other maturational factors (eg, increase in excitatory amino acid receptors and accompanying increased susceptibility to excitotoxic injury).

Evidence of metabolic impairment caused by deep hypothermic circulatory arrest also comes from studies of cerebral fractional oxygen extraction measured using NIRS. One report measured central venous saturation, derived fractional oxygen extraction, and found that subjects who had undergone deep hypothermic circulatory arrest had decreased fractional oxygen extraction during rewarming compared with subjects who had continuous flow during surgery [87]. This finding may relate to an impairment in cerebral oxygen metabolism after cooling that was demonstrated in other studies [88]. Hoffman and colleagues [89] also found cerebral oxygenation to be decreased after bypass and attributed these findings to increased cerebrovascular resistance after deep hypothermic bypass. Toet and colleagues [90] similarly found cerebral oxygenation to be diminished after bypass for up to 26 hours. These investigators performed neuropsychologic follow-up 30 to 36 months after surgery and found that only low cerebral oxygenation levels before surgery predicted abnormal follow-up testing.

In the postoperative period following cardiac surgery on bypass with hypothermic arrest, NIRS studies have demonstrated significant carbon dioxide vasoreactivity impairment for up to 48 hours [91]. In one study, carbon dioxide vasoreactivity was similar to a study of infants during hypothermic bypass [92], but was lower than in a study of ventilated term neonates [21]. There was a trend toward recovery of carbon dioxide vasoreactivity during the 48-hour study period. These data suggest a persistent impairment in vasoreactivity following bypass and hypothermic arrest. Combined with systemic instability that is common among postoperative neonates, this impairment of vasoreactivity could place these children at risk for cerebrovascular injury and subsequent neurologic impairment. The authors' research group found that elevated end-tidal CO_2 levels and high variability in mean arterial pressure were associated with pressure-passive cerebral perfusion, and, hence, a failure of the neonate to regulate cerebral oxyhemoglobin levels in the face of changing systemic pressure [93]. In this way, NIRS may be helpful in identifying those children with abnormal return of cerebrovascular regulatory capacity who are at increased risk for neurologic injury during postoperative disturbances in cardiorespiratory function.

Functional activation studies

Although NIRS has excellent temporal resolution, its spatial resolution is poor compared with imaging modalities, such as CT and MRI. Functional NIRS studies are based on the activation of a specific brain region as detected by localized hemodynamic responses (by NIRS) to specific motor, visual, or cognitive tasks. In adults, one study demonstrated that NIRS could determine language laterality reliably in healthy volunteers and subjects who had epilepsy [94]. Although studies of this nature are difficult to accomplish in newborns, Meek and colleagues [95] used NIRS to measure changes in oxyhemoglobin and deoxyhemoglobin over the occipital region in infants who were shown a visual stimulus. Infants who were shown a checkerboard pattern had increased oxyhemoglobin and deoxyhemoglobin levels compared with control infants.

Kusaka and colleagues [96] measured regional cerebral blood flow in the temporal lobes of infants who did and did not have neurologic abnormalities using NIRS with indocyanine green as an indicator. NIRS identified regions with abnormal blood flow that was due to hemorrhage as well as single photon emission computed tomography imaging.

Kotilahti and colleagues [97] showed that oxyhemoglobin concentration increased over the auditory cortices after auditory stimulation, and that the latency period between stimulation and oxygenation response decreased with gestational age. Zaramella and colleagues [98] found increased oxyhemoglobin concentrations and increased cerebral blood volume in the same region during auditory stimulation. Chen and colleagues [99] found that although normal term neonates showed increased oxyhemoglobin levels after auditory stimulation, neonates who had hypoxic-ischemic encephalopathy showed decreased total hemoglobin changes after auditory stimulation. Similarly, Taga and colleagues [100] demonstrated a significant increase in oxyhemoglobin concentrations over the occipital and prefrontal cortices after visual stimulation of neonates. In other studies, newborns demonstrated increased oxyhemoglobin concentrations over the orbitofrontal region when exposed to vanilla and colostrum [101], and a decrease in oxyhemoglobin in the same anatomic region when exposed to noxious smells (detergent and disinfectant) [102]. Similarly, Slater and colleagues [103] found that total hemoglobin concentrations increased significantly over the contralateral somatosensory cortex during heel pricks for blood draws. Demonstrating that motor cortex activity also can be imaged, Isobe and colleagues [104] demonstrated increased oxyhemoglobin levels in the contralateral primary sensorimotor areas among sedated newborns who were subjected to passive knee movement.

Limitations of near-infrared spectroscopy imaging

Pathlength measurements

Perhaps the most serious limitation of NIRS recordings is the difficulty in establishing the DPF. This was demonstrated in a study that measured DPF using phase-resolved spectroscopy in 283 subjects who ranged in age from 1 day to 50 years; the DPF increased with age but also varied significantly within age ranges [5]. Furthermore, certain pathologic processes, such as birth asphyxia, seemed to affect the DPF compared with healthy age-matched controls. Another study that compared NIRS with diffuse optical tomography found wide ranges in the values of chromophore concentrations [105]. The investigators reported that although NIRS could track changes in chromophore concentration, the technology was unable to measure absolute changes in chromophore concentration. Other studies have reported significant variance in absolute and relative chromophore concentrations when testing the reliability of NIRS [106–108]. This variability has impeded the establishment of normative data and reliable measurements of the absolute concentration of chromophores during recordings.

Time-of-flight devices and intensity-modulated devices increasingly have the capacity to measure pathlength for each wavelength used during the acquisition of data [109,110]. The capacity to calculate the DPF directly in a real-time manner during measurement would go a long way toward improving the reliability and validity of NIRS measurements and increasing the clinical usefulness of the technology.

Movement and light artifact

Measurement of NIRS signals requires that ambient light be blocked from the optodes to prevent contamination of the signals that are being measured. Usually, this is accomplished by using an opaque cloth. Movement, however, changes the interoptode distance, and produces artifactual signals. This is a significant problem in intrapartum fetal monitoring. Improvements in technology that filter artifactual signal would facilitate the use of this technology.

Summary

NIRS has the obvious advantage over other monitoring technologies because it allows noninvasive bedside measurement of cerebral hemodynamic variables using a portable device; however, it has been slow in entering routine clinical care for two principal reasons. First, technical limitations prevent NIRS devices from generating reliable absolute values for the concentration of measured chromophores. Therefore, clinicians cannot compare values between patients and cannot compare values that are measured at different sessions. Until NIRS is able to generate reliable absolute values, its usefulness is limited. Second, few large studies have evaluated the use of NIRS. Until these two limitations are addressed, it is likely that NIRS will remain almost exclusively a research instrument.

Conversely, the thoughtful and rational application of NIRS as a unique technology that allows for noninvasive continuous measurements of cerebral oxygenation and hemodynamics is likely to provide important insights into the complex interrelationships among physiologic and pathologic conditions that contribute to brain injury in sick newborn infants.

References

[1] Jobsis FF. Noninvasive, infrared monitoring of cerebral and myocardial oxygen sufficiency and circulatory parameters. Science 1977;198:1264–7.
[2] Brazy JE, Lewis DV, Mitnick MH, et al. Noninvasive monitoring of cerebral oxygenation in preterm infants: preliminary observations. Pediatrics 1985;75(2):217–25.
[3] Nicklin SE, Hassan IA, Wickramasinghe YA, et al. The light still shines, but not that brightly? The current status of perinatal near infrared spectroscopy. Arch Dis Child Fetal Neonatal Ed 2003;88(4):F263–8.
[4] Edwards AD, Brown GC, Cope M, et al. Quantification of concentration changes in neonatal human cerebral oxidized cytochrome oxidase. J Appl Physiol 1991;71(5):1907–13.
[5] Duncan A, Meek JH, Clemence M, et al. Measurement of cranial optical path length as a function of age using phase resolved near infrared spectroscopy. Pediatr Res 1996;39:889–94.
[6] Brown R, Wright G, Royston D. A comparison of two systems for assessing cerebral venous oxyhemoglobin saturation during cardiopulmonary bypass in humans. Anesthesia 1993;48(8):697–700.

[7] Wolf M, von Siebenthal K, Keel M, et al. Tissue oxygen saturation measured by near infrared spectrophotometry correlates with arterial oxygen saturation during induced oxygenation changes in neonates. Physiol Meas 2000;21(4):481–91.

[8] Chance B, Maris M, Sorge J, et al. A phase modulation system for dual wavelength difference spectroscopy of hemoglobin deoxygenation in tissue. Proceedings of the International Society for Optical Engineering 1990;1204:481–91.

[9] Watkin SL, Spencer SA, Dimmock PW, et al. A comparison of pulse oximetry and near infrared spectroscopy (NIRS) in the detection of hypoxaemia occurring with pauses in nasal airflow in neonates. J Clin Monit Comput 1999;15(7–8):441–7.

[10] Wyatt JS, Delpy DT, Cope M, et al. Quantification of cerebral oxygenation and hemodynamics in sick newborn infants by near infrared spectroscopy. Lancet 1986;2(8515):1063–6.

[11] Wyatt J, Cope M, Delpy D, et al. Quantitation of cerebral blood volume in newborn human infants by near infrared spectroscopy. J Appl Physiol 1990;68:1086–91.

[12] Wickramasinghe YA, Livera LN, Spencer SA, et al. Plethysmographic validation of near infrared spectroscopic monitoring of cerebral blood volume. Arch Dis Child 1992;67(4): 407–11.

[13] Edwards AD, Richardson C, Cope M, et al. Cotside measurement of cerebral blood flow in ill newborn infants by near infrared spectroscopy. Lancet 1988;2(8614):770–1.

[14] Patel J, Marks K, Roberts I, et al. Measurement of cerebral blood flow in newborn infants using near infrared spectroscopy with indocyanine green. Pediatr Res 1998;43(1): 34–9.

[15] Skov L, Pryds O, Greisen G. Estimating cerebral blood flow in newborn infants: comparison of near infrared spectroscopy and 133Xe clearance. Pediatr Res 1991;30(6):570–3.

[16] Bucher HU, Edwards AD, Lipp AE, et al. Comparison between near infrared spectroscopy and [133]Xenon clearance for estimation of cerebral blood flow in critically ill preterm infants. Pediatr Res 1993;33(1):56–60.

[17] Keller E, Nadler A, Alkadhi H, et al. Noninvasive measurement of regional cerebral blood flow and regional cerebral blood volume by near-infrared spectroscopy and indocyanine green dye dilution. Neuroimage 2003;20(2):828–39.

[18] Raabe A, Beck J, Gerlach R, et al. Near-infrared indocyanine green video angiography: a new method for intraoperative assessment of vascular flow. Neurosurgery 2003;52(1): 132–9.

[19] Yoxall CW, Weindling AM, Dawani NH, et al. Measurement of cerebral venous oxyhemoglobin saturation in children by near-infrared spectroscopy and partial jugular venous occlusion. Pediatr Res 1995;38(3):319–23.

[20] Kissack CM, Garr R, Wardle SP, et al. Cerebral fractional oxygen extraction is inversely correlated with oxygen delivery in the sick, newborn, preterm infant. J Cereb Blood Flow Metab 2005;25(5):545–53.

[21] Wyatt JS, Edwards AD, Cope M, et al. Response of cerebral blood volume to changes in arterial carbon dioxide tension in preterm and term infants. Pediatr Res 1991;29(6):553–7.

[22] Brun NC, Greisen G. Cerebrovascular response to carbon dioxide as detected by near-infrared spectroscopy: comparison of three different measures. Pediatr Res 1994;36(1): 20–4.

[23] Leung TS, Aladangady N, Elwell CE, et al. A new method for the measurement of cerebral blood volume and total circulating blood volume using near infrared spatially resolved spectroscopy and indocyanine green: application and validation in neonates. Pediatr Res 2004;55(1):134–41.

[24] Kissack CM, Garr R, Wardle SP, et al. Postnatal changes in cerebral oxygen extraction in the preterm infant are associated with intraventricular hemorrhage and hemorrhagic parenchymal infarction but not periventricular leukomalacia. Pediatr Res 2004;56(1):111–6.

[25] Wardle SP, Yoxall CW, Weindling AM. Determinants of cerebral fractional oxygen extraction using near infrared spectroscopy in preterm neonates. J Cereb Blood Flow Metab 2000; 20(2):272–9.

[26] Watzman HM, Kurth CD, Montenegro LM, et al. Arterial and venous contributions to near-infrared cerebral oximetry. Anesthesiology 2000;93(4):947–53.

[27] Vintzileos AM, Nioka S, Lake M, et al. Transabdominal fetal pulse oximetry with near-infrared spectroscopy. Am J Obstet Gynecol 2005;192(1):129–33.

[28] Kakogawa J, Sumimoto K, Ho E, et al. Transabdominal measurement of oxygenation of the placenta by near-infrared spectroscopy. Semin Thromb Hemost 2005;31(3): 297–301.

[29] Bennet L, Rossenrode S, Gunning MI, et al. The cardiovascular and cerebrovascular responses of the immature fetal sheep to acute umbilical cord occlusion. J Physiol 1999; 517(Pt 1):247–57.

[30] Bennet L, Roelfsema V, Pathipati P, et al. Relationship between evolving epileptiform activity and delayed loss of mitochondrial activity after asphyxia measured by near-infrared spectroscopy in preterm fetal sheep. J Physiol 2006;572(Pt 1):141–54.

[31] Newman JP, Peebles DM, Hanson MA. Adenosine produces changes in cerebral hemodynamics and metabolism as assessed by near-infrared spectroscopy in late-gestation fetal sheep in utero. Pediatr Res 2001;50(2):217–21.

[32] Peebles DM, Miller S, Newman JP, et al. The effect of systemic administration of lipopolysaccharide on cerebral haemodynamics and oxygenation in the 0.65 gestation ovine fetus in utero. BJOG 2003;110(8):735–43.

[33] Peebles DM, Edwards AD, Wyatt JS, et al. Changes in human fetal cerebral hemoglobin concentration and oxygenation during labor measured by near-infrared spectroscopy. Am J Obstet Gynecol 1992;166(5):624–8.

[34] Faris F, Doyle M, Wickramasinghe Y, et al. A non-invasive optical technique for intrapartum fetal monitoring: preliminary clinical studies. Med Eng Phys 1994;16(4): 287–91.

[35] Aldrich CJ, D'Antona D, Spencer JAD, et al. Late fetal heart decelerations and changes in cerebral oxygenation during the first stage of labour. Br J Obstet Gynaecol 1995;102(1): 9–13.

[36] Aldrich CJ, D'Antona D, Spencer JA, et al. Fetal heart rate changes and cerebral oxygenation measured by near-infrared spectroscopy during the first stage of labour. Eur J Obstet Gynecol Reprod Biol 1996;64(2):189–95.

[37] Hamilton RJ, O'Brien PM, Wickramasinghe YA, et al. Intrapartum fetal cerebral near infrared spectroscopy: apparent change in oxygenation demonstrated in a non viable fetus. Br J Obstet Gynaecol 1995;102(12):1004–7.

[38] Aldrich CJ, D'Antona D, Wyatt JS, et al. Fetal cerebral oxygenation measured by near-infrared spectroscopy shortly before birth and acid-base status at birth. Obstet Gynecol 1994;84(5):861–6.

[39] Seelbach-Gobel B. Correlation between NIR spectroscopy and pulse oximetry in the fetus. J Perinat Med 1996;24(1):69–75.

[40] Dietz V, Wolf M, Keel M, et al. CO_2 reactivity of the cerebral hemoglobin concentration in healthy term newborns measured by near infrared spectrophotometry. Biol Neonate 1999; 75(2):85–90.

[41] Weiss M, Dullenkopf A, Kolarova A, et al. Near-infrared spectroscopic cerebral oxygenation reading in neonates and infants is associated with central venous oxygen saturation. Paediatr Anaesth 2005;15(2):102–9.

[42] Shah AR, Kurth CD, Gwiazdowski SG, et al. Fluctuations in cerebral oxygenation and blood volume during endotracheal suctioning in premature infants. J Pediatr 1992; 120(5):769–74.

[43] Mosca FA, Colnaghi M, Lattanzio M, et al. Closed versus open endotracheal suctioning in preterm infants: effects on cerebral oxygenation and blood volume. Biol Neonate 1997; 72(1):9–14.

[44] Jenni OG, Wolf M, Hengartner M, et al. Impact of central, obstructive and mixed apnea on cerebral hemodynamics in preterm infants. Biol Neonate 1996;70(2):91–100.

[45] Urlesberger B, Kaspirek A, Pichler G, et al. Apnoea of prematurity and changes in cerebral oxygenation and cerebral blood volume. Neuropediatrics 1999;30(1):29–33.

[46] Yamamoto A, Yokoyama N, Yonetani M, et al. Evaluation of change of cerebral circulation by SpO_2 in preterm infants with apneic episodes using near infrared spectroscopy. Pediatr Int 2003;45(6):661–4.

[47] Livera LN, Spencer SA, Thorniley MS, et al. Effects of hypoxemia and bradycardia on neonatal cerebral hemodynamics. Arch Dis Child 1991;66:376–80.

[48] Pichler G, Urlesberger B, Muller W. Impact of bradycardia on cerebral oxygenation and cerebral blood volume during apnoea in preterm infants. Physiol Meas 2003;24(3): 671–80.

[49] Bucher HU, Wolf M, Keel M, et al. Effect of aminophylline on cerebral haemodynamics and oxidative metabolism in premature infants. Eur J Pediatr 1994;153(2):123–8.

[50] Dani C, Bertini G, Reali MF, et al. Brain hemodynamic changes in preterm infants after maintenance dose caffeine and aminophylline treatment. Biol Neonate 2000;78(1):27–32.

[51] Dani C, Bertini G, Pezzati M, et al. Brain hemodynamic effects of doxapram in preterm infants. Biol Neonate 2006;89(2):69–74.

[52] Edwards AD, Wyatt JS, Richardson C, et al. Effects of indomethacin on cerebral haemodynamics in very preterm infants. Lancet 1990;335(8704):1491–5.

[53] Liem KD, Hopman JC, Kollee LA, et al. Effects of repeated indomethacin administration on cerebral oxygenation and haemodynamics in preterm infants: combined near infrared spectrophotometry and Doppler ultrasound study. Eur J Pediatr 1994;153(7):504–9.

[54] Benders MJ, Dorrepaal CA, van de Bor M, et al. Acute effects of indomethacin on cerebral hemodynamics and oxygenation. Biol Neonate 1995;68(2):91–9.

[55] Patel J, Roberts I, Azzopardi D, et al. Randomized double-blind controlled trial comparing the effects of ibuprofen with indomethacin on cerebral hemodynamics in preterm infants with patent ductus arteriosus. Pediatr Res 2000;47(1):36–42.

[56] Volpe JJ. Hypoxic-ischemic encephalopathy: clinical aspects. In: Volpe JJ, editor. Neurology of the newborn. Philadelphia: W.B. Saunders Company; 2001. p. 331–94.

[57] Tyszczuk L, Meek J, Elwell C, et al. Cerebral blood flow is independent of mean arterial blood pressure in preterm infants undergoing intensive care. Pediatrics 1998;102(2 Pt 1): 337–41.

[58] Tsuji M, Saul JP, du Plessis A, et al. Cerebral intravascular oxygenation correlates with mean arterial pressure in critically ill premature infants. Pediatrics 2000;106(4):625–32.

[59] Soul JS, du Plessis AJ, Walter GL, et al. Near-infrared spectroscopy monitoring detects changes in cerebral blood flow in an animal model of acute hydrocephalus [abstract]. Ann Neurol 1998;44(3):535.

[60] Soul JS, Taylor GA, Wypij D, et al. Noninvasive detection of changes in cerebral blood flow by near-infrared spectroscopy in a piglet model of hydrocephalus. Pediatr Res 2000;48(4): 445–9.

[61] Munro MJ, Walker AM, Barfield CP. Hypotensive extremely low birth weight infants have reduced cerebral blood flow. Pediatrics 2004;114(6):1591–6.

[62] Pellicer A, Valverde E, Elorza MD, et al. Cardiovascular support for low birth weight infants and cerebral hemodynamics: a randomized, blinded, clinical trial. Pediatrics 2005; 115(6):1501–12.

[63] Lemmers PM, Toet M, van Schelven LJ, et al. Cerebral oxygenation and cerebral oxygen extraction in the preterm infant: the impact of respiratory distress syndrome. Exp Brain Res 2006 [Epub February 28, 2006].

[64] du Plessis A, Tsuji M, Naruse H, et al. Near infrared spectroscopy (NIRS) shows pronounced effects of CSF removal on cerebral hemodynamics in infantile hydrocephalus [abstract]. Pediatr Res 1995;37:377A.

[65] Casaer P, von Siebenthal K, van der Vlugt A, et al. Cytochrome aa3 and intracranial pressure in newborn infants; a near infrared spectroscopy study [letter]. Neuropediatrics 1992; 23(2):111.

[66] Soul JS, Eichenwald E, Walter G, et al. CSF removal in infantile posthemorrhagic hydro-cephalus results in significant improvement in cerebral hemodynamics. Pediatr Res 2004; 55(5):872–6.

[67] Schulz G, Keller E, Haensse D, et al. Slow blood sampling from an umbilical artery catheter prevents a decrease in cerebral oxygenation in the preterm newborn. Pediatrics 2003;111(1): e73–6.

[68] Roll C, Huning B, Kaunicke M, et al. Umbilical artery catheter blood sampling volume and velocity: impact on cerebral blood volume and oxygenation in very-low-birthweight infants. Acta Paediatr 2006;95(1):68–73.

[69] Baserga MC, Gregory GA, Sola A. Cerebrovascular response in small preterm infants during routine nursery gavage feedings. Biol Neonate 2003;83(1):12–8.

[70] Palmer K, Spencer SA, Wickramasinghe Y, et al. Negative extrathoracic pressure ventila-tion—evaluation of the neck seal. Early Hum Dev 1994;37(1):67–72.

[71] Kohlhauser C, Bernert G, Hermon M, et al. Effects of endotracheal suctioning in high-frequency oscillatory and conventionally ventilated low birth weight neonates on cerebral hemodynamics observed by near infrared spectroscopy (NIRS). Pediatr Pulmonol 2000; 29(4):270–5.

[72] Ramamoorthy C, Tabbutt S, Kurth CD, et al. Effects of inspired hypoxic and hypercapnic gas mixtures on cerebral oxygen saturation in neonates with univentricular heart defects. Anesthesiology 2002;96(2):283–8.

[73] Takami T, Yamamura H, Inai K, et al. Monitoring of cerebral oxygenation during hypoxic gas management in congenital heart disease with increased pulmonary blood flow. Pediatr Res 2005;58(3):521–4.

[74] Dorrepaal CA, Benders MJ, Steendijk P, et al. Cerebral hemodynamics and oxygenation in preterm infants after low-dose vs. high-dose surfactant replacement therapy. Biol Neonate 1993;64(4):193–200.

[75] Edwards AD, McCormick DC, Roth SC, et al. Cerebral hemodynamic effects of treatment with modified natural surfactant investigated by near infrared spectroscopy. Pediatr Res 1992;32(5):532–6.

[76] Roll C, Knief J, Horsch S, et al. Effect of surfactant administration on cerebral haemody-namics and oxygenation in premature infants—a near infrared spectroscopy study. Neuropediatrics 2000;31(1):16–23.

[77] van Bel F, Dorrepaal CA, Benders MJ, et al. Changes in cerebral hemodynamics and oxy-genation in the first 24 hours after birth asphyxia. Pediatrics 1993;92(3):365–72.

[78] Meek JH, Elwell CE, McCormick DC, et al. Abnormal cerebral haemodynamics in perina-tally asphyxiated neonates related to outcome. Arch Dis Child Fetal Neonatal Ed 1999; 81(2):F110–5.

[79] van Bel F, Shadid M, Moison RM, et al. Effect of allopurinol on postasphyxial free radical formation, cerebral hemodynamics, and electrical brain activity. Pediatrics 1998;101(2): 185–93.

[80] Toet MC, Lemmers PM, van Schelven LJ, et al. Cerebral oxygenation and electrical activity after birth asphyxia: their relation to outcome. Pediatrics 2006;117(2):333–9.

[81] Kurth CD, Steven JM, Nicolson SC, et al. Kinetics of cerebral deoxygenation dur-ing deep hypothermic circulatory arrest in neonates. Anesthesiology 1992;77(4): 656–61.

[82] du Plessis A, Newburger J, Jonas R, et al. Cerebral oxygen supply and utilization during infant cardiac surgery. Ann Neurol 1995;37:488–97.

[83] Kurth C, Steven J, Nicolson S. Cerebral oxygenation during pediatric cardiac surgery using deep hypothermic circulatory arrest. Anesthesiology 1995;82(1):74–82.

[84] Skov L, Greisen G. Apparent cerebral cytochrome aa3 reduction during cardio-pulmonary bypass in hypoxemic children with congenital heart disease. A critical analysis of in vivo near-infrared spectrophotometric data. Physiol Meas 1994;15(4): 447–57.

[85] Daubeney PEF, Pilkington SN, Janke E, et al. Cerebral oxygenation measured by near-in-frared spectroscopy: Comparison with jugular bulb oximetry. Ann Thorac Surg 1996;61(3): 930–4.

[86] Tortoriello TA, Stayer SA, Mott AR, et al. A noninvasive estimation of mixed venous ox-ygen saturation using near-infrared spectroscopy by cerebral oximetry in pediatric cardiac surgery patients. Paediatr Anaesth 2005;15(6):495–503.

[87] Wardle SP, Yoxall CW, Weindling AM. Cerebral oxygenation during cardiopulmonary bypass. Arch Dis Child 1998;78(1):26–32.

[88] Greeley WJ, Bracey VA, Ungerleider RM, et al. Recovery of cerebral metabolism and mi-tochondrial oxidation state is delayed after hypothermic circulatory arrest. Circulation 1991;84(5 Suppl):III400–6.

[89] Hoffman GM, Stuth EA, Jaquiss RD, et al. Changes in cerebral and somatic oxygenation during stage 1 palliation of hypoplastic left heart syndrome using continuous regional ce-rebral perfusion. J Thorac Cardiovasc Surg 2004;127(1):223–33.

[90] Toet MC, Flinterman A, Laar I, et al. Cerebral oxygen saturation and electrical brain ac-tivity before, during, and up to 36 hours after arterial switch procedure in neonates without pre-existing brain damage: its relationship to neurodevelopmental outcome. Exp Brain Res 2005;165(3):343–50.

[91] du Plessis AJ, Newburger J, Jonas RA, et al. Cerebral CO_2 vasoreactivity is impaired in the early postoperative period following hypothermic infant cardiac surgery [abstract]. Eur J Neurol 1995;2(Suppl 2):68A.

[92] Fallon P, Roberts I, Kirkham FJ, et al. Cerebral hemodynamics during cardiopulmonary bypass in children using near-infrared spectroscopy. Ann Thorac Surg 1993;56(6):1473–7.

[93] Bassan H, Gauvreau K, Newburger JW, et al. Identification of pressure passive cerebral perfusion and its mediators after infant cardiac surgery. Pediatr Res 2005;57(1):35–41.

[94] Watanabe E, Maki A, Kawaguchi F, et al. Non-invasive assessment of language dominance with near-infrared spectroscopic mapping. Neurosci Lett 1998;256(1):49–52.

[95] Meek JH, Firbank M, Elwell CE, et al. Regional hemodynamic responses to visual stimu-lation in awake infants. Pediatr Res 1998;43(6):840–3.

[96] Kusaka T, Isobe K, Nagano K, et al. Estimation of regional cerebral blood flow distribu-tion in infants by near-infrared topography using indocyanine green. Neuroimage 2001; 13(5):944–52.

[97] Kotilahti K, Nissila I, Huotilainen M, et al. Bilateral hemodynamic responses to auditory stimulation in newborn infants. Neuroreport 2005;16(12):1373–7.

[98] Zaramella P, Freato F, Amigoni A, et al. Brain auditory activation measured by near-infrared spectroscopy (NIRS) in neonates. Pediatr Res 2001;49(2):213–9.

[99] Chen S, Sakatani K, Lichty W, et al. Auditory-evoked cerebral oxygenation changes in hypoxic-ischemic encephalopathy of newborn infants monitored by near infrared spectros-copy. Early Hum Dev 2002;67(1–2):113–21.

[100] Taga G, Asakawa K, Hirasawa K, et al. Hemodynamic responses to visual stimulation in occipital and frontal cortex of newborn infants: a near-infrared optical topography study. Early Hum Dev 2003;75(Suppl 1):S203–10.

[101] Bartocci M, Winberg J, Ruggiero C, et al. Activation of olfactory cortex in newborn infants after odor stimulation: a functional near-infrared spectroscopy study. Pediatr Res 2000; 48(1):18–23.

[102] Bartocci M, Winberg J, Papendieck G, et al. Cerebral hemodynamic response to unpleasant odors in the preterm newborn measured by near-infrared spectroscopy. Pediatr Res 2001; 50(3):324–30.

[103] Slater R, Cantarella A, Gallella S, et al. Cortical pain responses in human infants. J Neuro-sci 2006;26(14):3662–6.

[104] Isobe K, Kusaka T, Nagano K, et al. Functional imaging of the brain in sedated newborn infants using near infrared topography during passive knee movement. Neurosci Lett 2001; 299(3):221–4.

[105] Boas DA, Gaudette T, Strangman G, et al. The accuracy of near infrared spectroscopy and imaging during focal changes in cerebral hemodynamics. Neuroimage 2001;13(1): 76–90.

[106] Menke J, Voss U, Moller G, et al. Reproducibility of cerebral near infrared spectroscopy in neonates. Biol Neonate 2003;83(1):6–11.

[107] Dullenkopf A, Kolarova A, Schulz G, et al. Reproducibility of cerebral oxygenation measurement in neonates and infants in the clinical setting using the NIRO 300 oximeter. Pediatr Crit Care Med 2005;6(3):344–7.

[108] Wolf M, von Siebenthal K, Keel M, et al. Comparison of three methods to measure absolute cerebral hemoglobin concentration in neonates by near-infrared spectrophotometry. J Biomed Opt 2002;7(2):221–7.

[109] Duncan A, Whitlock T, Cope M, et al. A multiwavelength, wideband, intensity-modulated spectrometer for near-IR spectroscopy and imaging. Proceedings of the International Society for Optical Engineering 1993;1888:248–57.

[110] Ijichi S, Kusaka T, Isobe K, et al. Developmental changes of optical properties in neonates determined by near-infrared time-resolved spectroscopy. Pediatr Res 2005;58(3):568–73.

ELSEVIER
SAUNDERS

CLINICS IN
PERINATOLOGY

Clin Perinatol 33 (2006) 729–744

Mass Spectrometry in Neonatal Medicine and Clinical Diagnostics—the Potential Use of Mass Spectrometry in Neonatal Brian Monitoring

Alan R. Spitzer, MD*, Donald Chace, PhD

Pediatrix Medical Group, 1301 Concord Terrace, Sunrise, FL 33323, USA

Mass spectrometry (MS) has had an important place in clinical chemistry and laboratory diagnostics for the past 4 decades. Historically, the value of MS was in its ability to measure the mass of bioactive metabolites (eg, amino acids, fatty acids, organic acids, steroids, lipids, neurotransmitters) in a selective, accurate, and comprehensive manner. Its primary use during this period was the organic acid analysis of urine for the diagnosis of metabolic abnormalities, and this capability remains one of its most important applications. Traditionally, most of these MS analyses were conducted in specialty, expert laboratories because the complex profiles produced by such devices required interpretation by experts in intermediary metabolism. In these applications, a mass spectrometer was often used in conjunction with a physical separation device (eg, gas chromatograph) to detect the mass of the intact molecule and its fragments. The fragmentation pattern uniquely identified a particular molecule that, when coupled to a retention time on a chromatographic device, was considered the gold standard in clinical analysis.

During the past 2 decades, the pharmaceutical industry, in an attempt to screen more rapidly for possible therapeutic efficacy, changed its approach to the discovery of new agents by evaluating many new compounds to find a single drug that might exert the desired pharmaceutical effect with a high margin of safety. The mass spectrometer became a critical tool in this screening process, and the increasing demand of the pharmaceutical companies led to the development of new mass measuring devices that could analyze polar compounds and higher molecular weight compounds more quickly, more accurately, and in larger numbers. The result of these efforts

---

* Corresponding author.

E-mail address: Alan_Spitzer@pediatrix.com (A.R. Spitzer).

0095-5108/06/$ - see front matter © 2006 Elsevier Inc. All rights reserved.
doi:10.1016/j.clp.2006.06.005   *perinatology.theclinics.com*

was the interface of liquid chromatography with MS for very polar or large molecules, such as peptides and proteins. The two techniques most often recognized in this field are actually ionization techniques (electrospray ionization and matrix-assisted laser desorption/ionization) that enabled metabolite/protein analysis for the largest variety of compounds possible. In fact, Nobel Prizes in chemistry were awarded recently to two mass spectrometrists for their work.

The history of MS in medicine is important because it clearly points to future applications. For example, one of the major goals of the pharmaceutical industry is to use screening to identify potential aberrations in the metabolism of their drugs during a clinical trial. Eliminating patients who might have a potentially adverse reaction to a particular drug because of a genetic variation in metabolism could improve the efficacy and safety of that drug. Alternatively, altering drug-dosing strategies because of that metabolic abnormality seems likely in the near future, and may soon herald an age of uniquely patient-specific approaches to medical treatment (therapeutic tailoring of care). In the areas of genetics and metabolism, one could also argue that basic substances of metabolism (eg, carbohydrates, amino acids, fatty acids) are subject to similar considerations because their metabolism can be affected if an individual has an abnormality in enzyme function. In fact, this approach was used for decades with organic acid analysis. However, basic organic acid analysis was not designed as a screening tool (ie, designed for large numbers of routine tests) and it was not indicated for the simple analysis of blood or plasma for metabolites (biomarkers) in unusually high concentrations. Furthermore, experts began questioning whether the biomarkers were present before a disease manifested and hence could predict whether a patient actually had a metabolic disease (or, in the pharmaceutical model, would experience an adverse event if given a particular drug).

The advent of neonatal screening

In the late 1980s and early 1990s, experts recognized the importance of carnitine and its fatty acid esters in mitochondrial metabolism, specifically beta-oxidation. Furthermore, whether these biomarkers were present appeared to be useful in detecting diseases of fatty acid or organic acid metabolism. Carnitine is a highly polar molecule, similar to amino acids, which can form esters with fatty acids called *acylcarnitines*. Carnitine and fatty acylcarnitine were not easily analyzed by the gas chromatograph/MS techniques available at that time. New techniques of MS, however, led to the development of methods that could readily detect these compounds. Information gathered from the analytic capability to detect carnitine and acylcarnitine led to further research into the importance of such biomarkers and their efficacy in detecting inherited disease in newborns. A specific type of mass spectrometer, a tandem mass spectrometer (tandem MS), was found to be especially useful because it could selectively detect and quantify many metabolites within a family of compounds, such as acylcarnitines and α-amino acids. This technique did not require chromatography (a time-consuming process) and could be performed using extracts of small quantities of blood, even including dried blood spots on cards of filter paper. This method, pioneered in the early 1990s, has undergone such substantial improvements in the area of sample preparation, data processing, and result interpretation that it is now considered a standard clinical tool in neonatal metabolic screening and metabolic disease assessment.

In addition to analyzing amino acids and acylcarnitines, tandem MS can be used to detect and evaluate the presence of many classes of metabolites, including steroids, bile acids, nucleic acids, fatty acids, and lipids. Most of these techniques, however, still require a chromatographic step or extensive sample purification and are therefore better suited for diagnostic testing and confirmation rather than screening. Rapid developments are on the horizon for new sample preparation systems and mass spectrometers that may be better suited for general population screening in these areas.

A mass spectrometry primer

Because MS is a tool, how it is used and what results can be expected must be understood. MS measures the mass of an electrically charged molecule known as an *ion* or *ionized molecule*. It can detect molecules ranging in size from mass values less than water (mass = 18) to greater than the mass of hemoglobin (mass = 66,980 g/mol). Charged molecules that have not been fragmented are known as *molecular ions* or *precursor ions*. Portions of molecules that have been fragmented are known as *fragment ions* or *product ions*. In a mass spectrometric analysis, results typically contain molecular ions, fragment ions, or both. Results produced by a mass spectrometer include the mass of the ion and the number of these ions. Often these data are displayed in a chart or graph called a *mass spectrum* (Figs. 1 and 2). The mass spectrum shows the mass value (along the *x* axis) and its quantity (along the *y* axis), often as bars or vertical lines. Typically, these data are simply represented in a database or spreadsheet format without the spectrum, or they are processed to produce a quantitative number (concentration). From the most common clinical chemistry perspective, the important outcome is to identify a compound (its presence at a particular mass) and its concentration (how large the peak is, or how much of that compound is present).

Clinical metabolomics

A closer look at the rapid expansion of newborn screening provides clues to the usefulness of MS in the newer applications of metabolomics and represents a model for future applications of screening in various diseases that

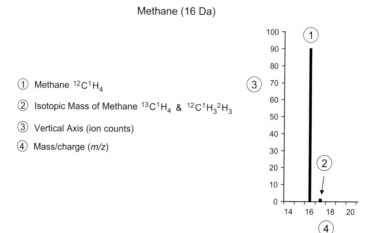

Fig. 1. Illustration of a mass spectrum of methane that would be obtained from electron ionization. The x axis is mass-to-charge ratio (m/z for mass identification) and the y axis is ion counts (for mass quantification). The monoisotopic mass of methane is 16 daltons (Da) and is the major peak in the spectrum. It is positioned at m/z 16 because the charge is 1. The natural isotopic contributions of a single carbon-13 or deuterium would be approximately 1.2%, and therefore a peak occurs at m/z 17.

affect neonates and adults. These diseases or metabolic abnormalities may result from one or a combination of factors in genetics, the environment, and nutrition. MS has changed the clinical chemistry/screening model from a single metabolite–single disease detection approach on a relatively large volume of blood to a multiple metabolite–multiple disease evaluation or panel on a much smaller sample of blood, often just a filter paper spot. In this case, a newborn screening panel might include measurement of several amino acids and numerous acylcarnitines. Specific amino acids, such as phenylalanine (Phe) or octanoylcarnitine (C8) (an eight-carbon saturated fatty acylcarnitine that is considered a medium-sized fatty acid), strongly correlate with the genetic diseases phenylketonuria (PKU) and medium-chain acyl-coA dehydrogenase (MCAD) deficiency, respectively. However, elevations of these metabolites could also represent transient abnormalities induced by intravenous alimentation with protein or the administration of drugs such as valproic acid. The clinical circumstances cannot be ignored when attempting to make an appropriate diagnosis with tandem MS.

At first glance in the specific cases of PKU or MCAD deficiency, a single diagnostic metabolite appears to be all clinicians must be concerned about. However, several other metabolites are often characteristic of a specific disease state or environmental factor. In PKU, for example, the amino acid tyrosine (Tyr) is also critical in accurate screening for this disease (Fig. 3). Its simultaneous measurement by tandem MS permits the calculation of the Phe/Tyr ratio, a well-known index for accurate identification of PKU.

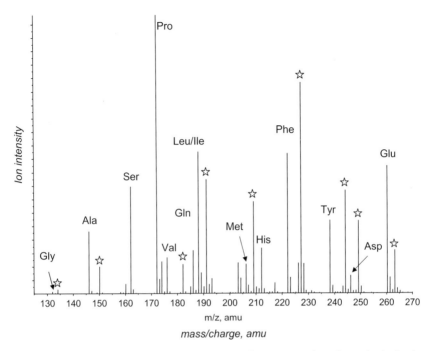

Fig. 2. Tandem mass spectra of dried blood extracts from a normal newborn obtained using neutral loss (NL) of 102-Da scan that detects α-amino acids. The stars represent isotopically labeled amino acids used as reference standards. Ala, alanine; amu, atomic mass unit; Asp, aspartic acid; Gln, glutamine; Glu, glutamic acid; Gly, glycine; His, histidine; Ile, isoleucine; Leu, leucine; Met, methionine; Phe, phenylalanine; Ser, serine; Tyr, tyrosine; Val, valine.

Knowledge of metabolic pathways would show that the conversion of Phe to Tyr is deficient in PKU, and therefore Phe levels would be expected to elevate and those of Tyr to decline. Consequently, the ratio would increase more rapidly than the elevation of Phe levels alone. With parenteral nutrition, however, the profile that emerges in some infants should be somewhat different. Because the conversion of Phe to Tyr is normal, an abnormal ratio would not be expected, even though elevations of Phe might be seen. Because most total parenteral nutrition (TPN) solutions also contain Tyr, these levels are expected to be more elevated than in PKU (Fig. 4).

With MCAD deficiency, C8 represents the key diagnostic indicator, but important biomarkers are altered by the enzyme deficiency, including 6- and 10-carbon (saturated and unsaturated) acylcarnitine species. As a result, detection of MCAD deficiency is based partly on a generalized pattern or profile of these elevated acylcarnitines. Furthermore, fatty acids, which are present in abundance, bind with available free carnitine and are eliminated in urine and bile. This process can result in a secondary carnitine deficiency, but also permits the calculation of a ratio of C8 to free carnitine.

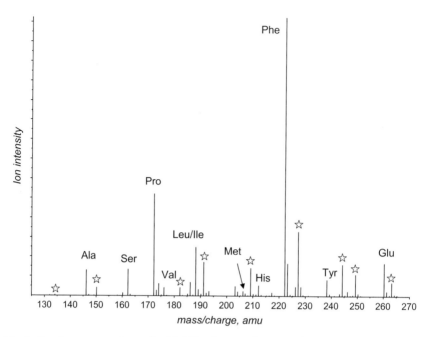

Fig. 3. Tandem mass spectrum of a dried blood extract from a newborn with phenylketonuria. Note the elevation of phenylalanine relative to the internal standard and the slight decrease in the concentration of tyrosine. Ala, alanine; amu, atomic mass unit; Asp, aspartic acid; Gln, glutamine; Glu, glutamic acid; Gly, glycine; His, histidine; Ile, isoleucine; Leu, leucine; Met, methionine; Phe, phenylalanine; Ser, serine; Tyr, tyrosine; Val, valine.

Ratios may also be helpful in detecting the administration of valproate or medium-chain triglyceride (MCT) oil. The unsaturated fatty acylcarnitine is not seen in valproate or MCT oil metabolism, but is seen in MCAD deficiency. Hence, the ratio of C10/C10:1 may be helpful in differentiating MCAD from other causes of these metabolite elevations.

Using this approach, tandem MS has measured as many as 65 diagnostic metabolites and ratios. Most importantly, however, is that this analysis can be performed using a blood spot on filter paper, potentially assessing many diseases in a single analysis from one blood spot. Two things are important to note. By measuring multiple metabolites, the cost of screening screen per disease is reduced and greater amounts of information are provided that may be valuable in differentiating genetic or environmental causes of metabolite elevations. In addition, this approach reduces the likelihood of false results through improved pattern recognition, and the patterns can be readily expanded as new validations of metabolites in screening are achieved. Because the analysis is based on a blood spot dried onto filter paper, the hazards of working with liquid biologic fluids are decreased and shipping costs are reduced because blood spots can be mailed in an envelope and do not need to be sent in a large box packed with dry ice.

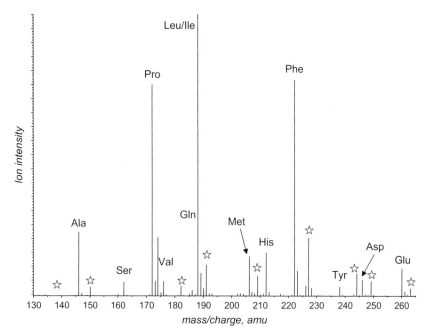

Fig. 4. Tandem mass spectrum of a dried blood extract from a premature infant on total parenteral nutrition (TPN). Note the elevations of Phe, leucine, and methionine relative to their internal standards. Also note the decrease in the concentration of Tyr. TPN profiles may or may not
have elevated Tyr, depending on the formulation. Ala, alanine; amu, atomic mass unit; Asp, aspartic acid; Gln, glutamine; Glu, glutamic acid; Gly, glycine; His, histidine; Ile, isoleucine; Leu,
leucine; Met, methionine; Phe, phenylalanine; Ser, serine; Tyr, tyrosine; Val, valine.

Road map to diagnosis

Medicine is not always characterized by clear-cut diagnostics based on
clinical laboratory tests. This fact is partly because the focus traditionally relies on results of individual tests and other diagnostic indicators in an un-
healthy state. What about these indicators in a healthy state? For example,
MCAD deficiency is well-known to be undiagnosable without a standard
clinical chemistry test until a child becomes severely hypoglycemic, often comatose, and occasionally presents in a severely debilitated, preterminal condition. What is important, however, is that the critical metabolites in MCAD
are present in the well state and the disease state. In metabolism and metabolic screening, the identifiable metabolic patterns that indicate a disease
must be detectable before the disease becomes manifest. Although these metabolites may not always be easy to interpret or obvious, they are apparent to
the trained eye and are highly predictive of future problems if left untreated.

The analogy of metabolism to a road map is actually quite appropriate.
For example, if an accident occurs on a major freeway, both the traffic intensity and alternative routes would determine whether automobiles reach

their destinations, and whether these automobiles affect other roads. When a severe accident occurs at rush hour, traffic backs up very quickly. Cars will not be able to enter the highway ahead of the obstructed road, and many cars will look for alternative routes. The alternative routes typically will be used more heavily than normal, creating other backups along these routes. If the traffic jam is not freed, these routes will expand so that surrounding business may be affected and may even have to close if employees cannot get to work. How similar circumstances can arise with metabolites is easy to imagine. With a metabolic disease, the major pathway of metabolism is blocked and the alternative routes become activated. Many of these routes have adverse effects as certain biochemicals build up, because they were not meant to be so "heavily traveled" (ie, toxic metabolites can be handled efficiently at the normal lower concentrations, but not at these suddenly emerging new levels).

With metabolism or MCAD deficiency, for example, as long as the alternative pathways have enough capacity, no disease may be detected. Conversely, if a major event occurs in which the normal elimination of metabolites is suddenly obstructed on the metabolic highway, backups and traffic jams occur. This circumstance is analogous to what is observed during drug treatments or TPN. What is often unknown, however, is what level of traffic the highway can tolerate, which is where individual variation occurs and why simply monitoring the traffic under various clinical circumstances may be important.

Finally, in some cases, the carriers and environment are what are most interesting. What about a highway system on which heavy construction is occurring, where one lane is closed and backups occur primarily during rush hour? In this instance, the traffic is not persistent and the untoward effects are temporary. The alternative routes are well planned with no undesired effects. But what if a problem occurs (another genetic abnormality or partial abnormality) in a minor pathway? A multiple carrier or related disease could present a problem that is still detectable based on metabolism, but not on the specific gene alone. This scenario is the primary advantage and challenge of metabolic screening.

This field will also clearly introduce greater integration and measurement of defective enzymes in the future. MS may enable detection of the abnormal enzyme (a protein) compared with the normal one. Proteomics and MS are just entering the clinical world of diagnostics and screening.

Proteomics and genomics in the diagnosis of neonatal–perinatal disease

In areas of biomarker discovery, MS has played a key role. New proteins or compounds are commonly being characterized partly through MS. One could naturally assume that this same technology could detect the compounds in various bodily fluids or tissues on a routine clinical basis. However, various challenges still need to be overcome for MS to be a robust, easy-to-use, inexpensive tool for routine, high-volume protein analysis. Currently, the primary difficulty in measuring the concentrations of interesting proteins in plasma or blood is the presence of the major blood proteins such as hemoglobin or albumin. Extensive sample preparation and purification are needed to isolate that needle in the haystack. Many scientists are working toward these more highly automated systems, but this still requires much work on the systems, not mass spectrometers, to isolate and purify proteins that may serve as relevant biomarkers. Furthermore, even with advanced sample preparation systems, the quantity of resulting data can be overwhelming and difficult to interpret. Equally important to the developments of analytic systems for proteomics are the information systems (informatics) that are required.

Currently, mass spectrometers are primarily used to identify new biomarkers and better understand the role of proteins. Once identified, these markers are detected by simpler, often less-specific techniques and then reconfirmed by mass spectrometer. It is just a matter of time before the technology advances sufficiently for protein analysis by MS to become as routine as a newborn screening test.

Genomic assessment, however, may be more appropriate for other technologies and other circumstances. Although the unraveling of the human genome in recent years has been understandably viewed as one of the great advances in scientific achievement, one must remember that the genetic potential of an individual is different from the expression of that potential during a specific clinical situation. Identifying the presence of a certain gene, for example, only shows that the individual has that gene and a potential for a disease to become manifest in the future. It does not indicate, however, whether that gene may ever express itself clinically (especially true of the heterozygous state), to what extent it may express, and whether the expression will result in sufficient pathophysiology to result in a clear clinical abnormality. On the other hand, MS detection of abnormal metabolites or biomarkers in the blood is far more likely to result from the initiation of a disease or disease process. The future will likely require an understanding of genetic potential for disease (or abnormality in metabolism, such as with certain drugs) and a methodology for detecting appropriate biomarkers in the blood during early stages of a disease, so that intervention can ideally prevent the full manifestation of the disease process and thereby limit morbidity.

Mass spectrometers have been used to identify proteins and metabolic biomarkers in batch analysis. The ability to measure the mass of these compounds makes for a very accurate analysis. However, although the technology available to molecular biologists allows them to identify gene fragments without needing a mass spectrometer, identification of their expression is important. Therefore, the advantage of mass spectrometer in genetics and single nucleotide polymorphism analysis may more appropriately be the ability to multiplex without the need for extensive probes. Perhaps with enhanced sensitivity, a mass spectrometer will be able to measure the gene fragments directly.

Neonatal brain monitoring—causes of neonatal brain injury

No aspect of neonatal outcome is more critical than brain function throughout life. As neonatal medicine evolved as a specialty during the latter part of the 20th century, it went through a series of critical stages, especially regarding very low birth weight (VLBW) infants. Initially, the great challenge was to refine therapy to the point where these infants could survive. Once they began to survive in sufficient numbers, the associated morbidities of care (eg, bronchopulmonary dysplasia, necrotizing enterocolitis, the patent ductus arteriosus) emerged as focal points of clinical research. Ultimately, the quality of life for these neonates, determined greatly by long-term neurodevelopmental outcome, became the question of greatest importance. Because no aspect of life defines the human being as specifically as brain function and ability, the importance of understanding the causes of neonatal brain injury and its prevention has become paramount.

The primary methods of assessing brain injury in the neonatal period currently involve some aspect of brain imaging. Cranial ultrasound, CT, and MRI of various types (eg, magnetic resonance angiography, magnetic resonance spectroscopy, diffusion-weighted imaging) [1–4] have been the tools used to define the extent of injury during the neonatal period and the likelihood of permanent injury after discharge from the neonatal intensive care unit (NICU). More recently, other interesting techniques, such as cerebral function monitoring (CFM), have been used to examine neonatal brain development and neurologic injury [5,6]. Initially, neonatal brain hemorrhage was believed to have the greatest long-term consequence for VLBW babies [7]. In more recent years, white matter disease (WMD) and periventricular leukomalacia (PVL), believed to be alternative and related expressions of chronic hypoxic-ischemic injury in the neonate, have attracted attention as the events most likely to produce more permanent neurologic disability in the form of cerebral palsy and developmental delay [8]. In the term infant, hypoxic-ischemic injury and birth trauma seem to be more significant events in the evolution of brain injury [9]. Experts have widely recognized, however, that although many neonates who ultimately develop cerebral palsy sustain their injury during birth or in the NICU, some do not have any evidence of acute neonatal events capable of producing permanent injury [10–12].

When injury in the VLBW and term infant does not appear to be the result of some aspect of neonatal or perinatal care, the obvious question is, when does it occur? Since the early 1990s, it has become increasingly apparent that some perinatal brain injury is probably initiated before the neonatologist ever sees the patient. In examining the factors that resulted in preterm labor, Romero and colleagues [13,14] began to notice that certain prostaglandins appeared elevated in mothers delivering prematurely [13,14]. They speculated that preterm labor may be the result of an inflammatory process, with intrauterine infection the most likely cause of inflammation. This infection may not be clinically apparent, and many women may have subclinical chorioamnionitis, which goes entirely unrecognized until premature labor ensues. More importantly, the amniotic fluid of mothers of infants who developed cerebral palsy showed significant elevations of cytokines that were not increased in neonates who did not develop cerebral palsy [15,16]. Although this finding was comforting to neonatologists who often agonized over what may have caused their patient to sustain white matter injury, even when no clear-cut events in the NICU were observed, it made the diagnosis of maternal infection and inflammation that much more important. Numerous studies have confirmed these initial observations [17]. Furthermore, researchers also recognized that bronchopulmonary dysplasia, as an inflammatory process in the lung, probably had a similar onset before birth and was later aggravated by various commonplace events in the NICU [18]. Consequently, the diagnosis of maternal inflammatory disease now occupies a central role in neonatal–perinatal research, and the specific timing of the onset of infection has become increasingly important. Lastly, the possibility of early diagnosis of intrauterine infection as a more treatable entity has emerged as a critical focus of perinatal investigation. But an important question remains: if the disease process is often subclinical, how can it be easily detected?

Diagnosing neonatal sepsis remains a major challenge in newborn medicine, further demonstrating the difficulty of diagnosing intrauterine sepsis. Although presumed or suspected sepsis is the most common admitting diagnosis to the NICU, no foolproof diagnostic method is available. Many infants who appear to have clinical septicemia often yield negative blood cultures, which are the current gold standard for diagnosis. Because of the absence of any confirmatory test (C-reactive protein is helpful, but less diagnostic than a blood culture, as are white blood cell counts), many babies are treated with antibiotics for prolonged periods, probably unnecessarily [19]. In addition, prolonged antibiotic use is well-known to breed resistance microorganisms, which is an ever-present danger for NICU infants.

At the same time the etiologic factors of white matter injury in the VLBW infant were being examined, new attention began to focus on the term neonate with hypoxic-ischemic encephalopathy. Few problems have been as troubling to the perinatologist and neonatologist as birth asphyxia. Because so many of these infants ultimately either die or experience permanent neurologic injury, and because so many of these cases ultimately result in malpractice litigation, physicians are desperate to understand the origins of this entity. Even the diagnosis has been an ongoing concern, and the American College of Obstetrics and Gynecology and the American Academy of Pediatrics have labored repeatedly to better categorize this entity and the factors that result in an asphyxiated infant. However, the primary motivation for the increased interest in rapid diagnosis of perinatal hypoxic-ischemic injury was the recognition that brain and body cooling seemed to limit the manifestations of the disease process [20,21]. However, the initiation of brain and body hypothermia seemed to be required before 6 hours of life to discern any beneficial effect. Later application seemed to have little, if any, value for the asphyxiated infant.

Several trials have confirmed the benefit of hypothermia after perinatal hypoxic-ischemic injury [22,23]. Of concern, however, is that the overall results have not been as dramatic as originally anticipated. In examining the results, many clinicians have observed that the most significant variable over which little control could be exerted is the time between the onset of intrauterine hypoxemia and the time of birth. As with the VLBW baby and the development of WMD, one of the principal problems encountered in these trials was the inability to accurately determine the period during which the infant was initially becoming asphyxiated in utero. If a technique could be developed to provide this information, cooling would seem to be far more likely to influence outcome.

Lastly, although much neurologic injury has rightly been attributed to the extremely stressful events encountered by the fetus and neonate in the intrauterine environment and the NICU, other factors probably also influence long-term outcome in ways that are not yet apparent. Optimal neonatal nutrition, for example, remains an ongoing puzzle and a major concern. Researchers have noted that the extremely low birth weight (ELBW) neonate shows a form of "failure-to-thrive" in the NICU, with growth rates far below intrauterine accretion of protein and weight gain [24]. In effort to overcome this form of malnutrition, many neonatologists provide high levels of protein through a combination of intravenous alimentation and enteral feeding. The intravenous solutions of protein that are typically used in the NICU are the same ones used in adults, but the ability of the ELBW baby to metabolize the amino acids have not been tested in large numbers of these infants. Given the history of problems with excessive protein administration in newborn infants, the administration of high protein concentrations may overwhelm the enzymatic capacity of the ELBW baby to successfully metabolize these amino acids. This therapy may result in levels of certain amino acids such as phenylalanine and metabolic byproducts that produce temporary but important toxicities (Fig. 4). These toxicities, especially if unrecognized, may be one reason why some infants who do not experience typical types of injury, such as intraventricular hemorrhage (IVH) and periventricular leukomalacia (PVL), still may have poorer long-term outcomes than expected.

Metabolic brain monitoring by mass spectroscopy during the neonatal period

Although imaging studies have been extraordinarily valuable in detecting perinatal events and brain injury, by the time an infant shows an altered appearance of the brain, significant changes have already occurred. Extensive alterations in brain metabolism have already occurred by the time events such as IVH or PVL can be radiographically observed. Ideally, one would prefer to have a diagnostic tool that reflects altered metabolism at a point when the injury has not yet occurred and when intervention may lead to a highly improved outcome. MS appears to provide such possibilities.

The current literature on neonatal MS as a diagnostic tool is limited to neonatal screening for metabolic disorders. Currently, more than 50 metabolic diseases can be diagnosed using this technique. Most importantly, the technology seems ideally suited to the needs of the neonate. Because so many metabolites or biologic markers can be determined with a very small volume of blood (essentially a drop or two on filter paper), much information can be determined with minimal stress to the infant and studies are much easier to perform repeatedly, because blood loss is minimized. Furthermore, the technique may also be advantageous in the high-risk pregnancy. Screening of maternal blood and amniotic fluid would appear to offer ideal sources for examining metabolites, proteins, and other biomarkers that may indicate ongoing problems with a pregnancy before they manifest clinically.

In fact, initial studies strongly suggest the value of this technology in monitoring pregnancy and neonatal care. Using surface-enhanced laser desorption/time-of-flight spectroscopy, Gravett and colleagues [25] identified intra-amniotic infection (IAI) through proteomic profiling of novel biomarkers in rhesus monkeys and women who experienced preterm labor (Fig. 5), successfully showing unique protein expression profiles. In particular, calgranulin B and some novel immunoregulators appeared to be overexpressed in amniotic fluid and blood. They speculated that the ability to diagnose these biomarkers may ultimately lead to early detection of IAI and interventions that could improve outcome. This work was recently confirmed by Ruetschi and colleagues [26], who found overexpression of 17 proteins in amniotic fluid more commonly in women who experienced preterm labor than those who experienced ruptured membranes. Furthermore, early detection of congenital abnormalities through similar techniques seems to be on the immediate horizon. The potential changes in the approach to pregnancy that these studies portend cannot be overemphasized.

In the neonatal period, less work has been done in the area of proteomics and metabolomics, but studies are underway that may have a similar impact on the neonate. Although many studies have examined specific cytokines in WMD and PVL, the application of MS and identification of novel biomarkers have been minimal. However, very promising work is proceeding rapidly in related fields of medicine. Adult traumatic brain injury has been studied and novel biomarkers that appear to be specific to trauma have been identified, providing a new technique for following the evolution of such injuries [27]. In Alzheimer's disease, cerebrospinal fluid has also been found to contain specific biomarkers that may herald the disease and assist in charting its progress [28,29]. Other disease entities of adults, such as Parkinson's and other neurodegenerative disorders, have also been active areas of proteomic research, although this avenue of investigation is still in the

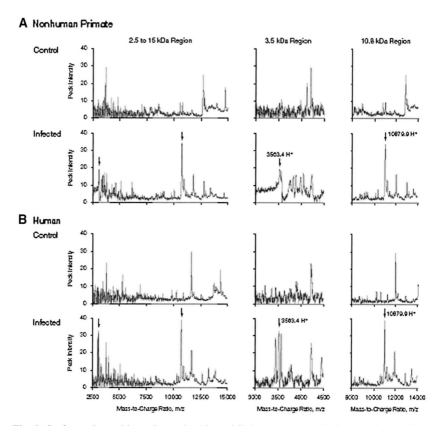

Fig. 5. Surface-enhanced laser desorption/time-of-flight spectroscopy indicates enhanced laser desorption/ionization time of flight. Group B *Streptococcus* infection induced differential protein expression in primate (*A*) and human (*B*) amniotic fluid samples. Detailed spectra show increased expression of the 3.5-kDa and 10.8-kDa peaks between control and infection. Arrows indicate unique peaks represented by polypeptides overexpressed in infection. (*From* Gravett MG, Novy MJ, Rosenfeld RG, et al. Diagnosis of intraamniotic infection by protein profiling and identification of novel biomarkers. JAMA 2004;292:462–9, with permission.)

early stages [30]. The application of similar approaches to neonatal brain injury seems imminent, although the path ahead will certainly not be straightforward. Our group at Pediatrix Medical Group has initiated a series of studies to examine the metabolomics of protein administration in ELBW neonates. We are also considering animal model studies on various mechanisms of brain injury in the neonatal period.

Because the results of obstetrical and neonatal studies are currently so minimal, few comments can be made about the likely success of present interventions (eg, early treatment of intrauterine infection with antibiotics, early delivery of potentially asphyxiated infants) or whether new types of interventions will emerge. Few areas of investigation, however, seem to offer as much promise in understanding and preventing neonatal brain injury as proteomics and metabolomics. As clinical tests using MS become more numerous, the ability to measure (1) multiple biomarkers in a single analysis, (2) metabolites from small volumes of biological fluids in a dried blood spot, and (3) a specific chemical attribute mass lends itself to a highly accurate, sensitive, and selective analysis. Furthermore, because the process can be automated and large samples can be run, neonatal physicians will most certainly encounter this technology with increasing frequency in the very near future.

References

[1] Burdjalov V, Srinivasan P, Baumgart S, et al. Handheld, portable ultrasound in the neonatal intensive care nursery: a new, inexpensive tool for the rapid diagnosis of common neonatal problems. J Perinatol 2002;22(6):478–83.

[2] Husain AM, Smergel E, Legido A, et al. Comparison of MRI and MRA findings in children with a variety of neurologic conditions. Pediatr Neurol 2000;23(4):307–11.

[3] Vigneron DB. Magnetic resonance spectroscopic imaging of human brain development. Neuroimaging Clin N Am 2006;16(1):75–85.

[4] Counsell SJ, Shen Y, Boardman JP, et al. Axial and radial diffusivity in preterm infants who have diffuse white matter changes on magnetic resonance imaging at term-equivalent age. Pediatrics 2006;117(2):376–86.

[5] Burdjalov VF, Baumgart S, Spitzer AR. Cerebral Function Monitoring—a new scoring system for the evaluation of brain maturation in neonates. Pediatrics 2003;112:855–61.

[6] West CR, Groves AM, Williams CE, et al. Early low cardiac output is associated with compromised electroencephalographic activity in very preterm infants. Pediatr Res 2006; 59(4):610–5.

[7] Papile LA, Burstein J, Burstein R, et al. Incidence and evolution of subependymal and intraventricular hemorrhage: a study of infants with birth weights less than 1,500 gm. J Pediatr 1978;92:529–34.

[8] Volpe JJ. Cerebral white matter injury of the premature infant—more common than you think. Pediatrics 2003;112(pt. 1):176–80.

[9] Berger R, Garnier Y. Perinatal brain injury. J Perinat Med 2000;28(4):261–85.

[10] Tran U, Gray PH, O'Callaghan MJ. Neonatal antecedents for cerebral palsy in extremely preterm babies and interaction with maternal factors. Early Hum Dev 2005;81(6):555–61.

[11] Laptook AR, O'Shea TM, Shankaran S, et al. Adverse neurodevelopmental outcomes among extremely low birth weight infants with a normal head ultrasound: prevalence and antecedents. Pediatrics 2005;115(3):673–80.

[12] Wood NS, Costeloe K, Gibson AT, et al. The EPICure study: associations and antecedents of neurological and developmental disability at 30 months of age following extremely preterm birth. Arch Dis Child Fetal Neonatal Ed 2005;90(2):F134–40.

[13] Romero R, Parvizi ST, Oyarzun E, et al. Amniotic fluid interleukin-1 in spontaneous labor at term. J Reprod Med 1990;35(3):235–8.

[14] Romero R, Avila C, Santhanam U, et al. Amniotic fluid interleukin 6 in preterm labor. Association with infection. J Clin Invest 1990;85(5):1392–400.

[15] Yoon BH, Romero R, Yang SH, et al. Interleukin-6 concentrations in umbilical cord plasma are elevated in neonates with white matter lesions associated with periventricular leukomalacia. Am J Obstet Gynecol 1996;174(5):1433–40.

[16] Yoon BH, Jun JK, Romero R, et al. Amniotic fluid inflammatory cytokines (interleukin-6, interleukin-1beta, and tumor necrosis factor-alpha), neonatal brain white matter lesions, and cerebral palsy. Am J Obstet Gynecol 1997;177(1):19–26.

[17] Ellison VJ, Mocatta TJ, Winterbourn CC, et al. The relationship of CSF and plasma cytokine levels to cerebral white matter injury in the premature newborn. Pediatr Res 2005;57(2):282–6.

[18] Dammann O, Leviton A, Bartels DB, et al. Lung and brain damage in preterm newborns. Are they related? How? Why? Biol Neonate 2004;85(4):305–13.

[19] Spitzer AR, Kirkby S, Kornhauser M. Practice variation in neonatal sepsis—a costly problem in newborn intensive care. J Perinatol 2005;25:265–9.

[20] Bona E, Hagberg H, Loberg EM, et al. Protective effects of moderate hypothermia after neonatal hypoxia-ischemia: short- and long-term outcome. Pediatr Res 1998;43(6):738–45.

[21] Gunn AJ, Gluckman PD, Gunn TR. Selective head cooling in newborn infants after perinatal asphyxia: a safety study. Pediatrics 1998;102(4 Pt 1):885–92.

[22] Gluckman PD, Wyatt JS, Azzopardi D, et al. Selective head cooling with mild systemic hypothermia after neonatal encephalopathy: multicentre randomised trial. Lancet 2005; 365(9460):663–70.

[23] Shankaran S, Laptook AR, Ehrenkranz RA, et al. Whole-body hypothermia for neonates with hypoxic-ischemic encephalopathy. N Engl J Med 2005;353(15):1574–84.

[24] Clark RH, Wagner CL, Merritt RJ, et al. Nutrition in the neonatal intensive care unit: how do we reduce the incidence of extrauterine growth restriction? J Perinatol 2003;23(4):337–44.

[25] Gravett MG, Novy MJ, Rosenfeld RG, et al. Diagnosis of intra-amniotic infection by proteomic profiling and identification of novel biomarkers. JAMA 2004;292(4):462–9.

[26] Ruetschi U, Rosen A, Karlsson G, et al. Proteomic analysis using protein chips to detect biomarkers in cervical and amniotic fluid in women with intra-amniotic inflammation. J Proteome Res 2005;4(6):2236–42.

[27] Haskins WE, Kobeissy FH, Wolper RA, et al. Rapid discovery of putative protein biomarkers of traumatic brain injury by SDS-PAGE-capillary liquid chromatography-tandem mass spectrometry. J Neurotrauma 2005;22(6):629–44.

[28] Selle H, Lamerz J, Buerger K, et al. Identification of novel biomarker candidates by differential peptidomics analysis of cerebrospinal fluid in Alzheimer's disease. Comb Chem High Throughput Screen 2005;8(8):801–6.

[29] Lopez MF, Mikulskis A, Kuzdzal S, et al. High-resolution serum proteomic profiling of Alzheimer disease samples reveals disease-specific, carrier-protein-bound mass signatures. Clin Chem 2005;51(10):1946–54.

[30] Fonteh AN, Harrington RJ, Huhmer AF, et al. Identification of disease markers in human cerebrospinal fluid using lipidomic and proteomic methods. Dis Markers 2006;22(1–2): 39–64.

ELSEVIER
SAUNDERS

CLINICS IN
PERINATOLOGY

Clin Perinatol 33 (2006) 745–750

Index

Note: Page numbers of article titles are in **boldface** type.

A

Acidosis
  amplitude-integrated EEG in, 641
  in hypercapnia, 586

Acylcarnitines, mass spectrometric
  detection of, 730–736

Aminophylline, cerebral oxygenation
  changes due to, 715

Amplitude-integrated
  electroencephalography, **619–632**
  advantages of, 620–621, 661–662
  background pattern in, 595–597,
    606–607, 621–625
  blood pressure effects on, 640–641
  classification of patterns in, 602–608,
    621–622
  disadvantages of, 662
  gestational age and, 595–596, 602–603
  historical review of, 594–595
  in acute metabolic failure, 597–598
  in carbon dioxide abnormalities, 641
  in compromised brain function,
    603–605
  in full-term newborn, **619–632**
  in hypoglycemia, 641
  in intensive care, 641–642
  in intraventricular hemorrhage,
    637–638
  in ischemia monitoring, 614
  in patent ductus arteriosus, 641
  in preterm infants, **633–647**
  in seizures, 598–601, 661–662
  in sleep–wake cycle, 606, 635–637
  in white matter injury, 637–638
  limitations of, 595
  medication effects on, 638–640
  normal, 596–597, 602–603, 634–635
  practical aspects of, 642–643
  principles of, 594–595, 620
  prognostic value of, 622–625
  publications on, 668–669
  seizure detection in, 625–627
  single-channel versus multiple-
    channel, 672, 674
  training for, **667–677**

  versus standard EEG, 593–594, 622

Antiepileptic drugs, for seizures, 658–660

Apnea
  drugs for, cerebral oxygenation
    changes due to, 715
  monitoring of, 613

Apoptosis, in cerebral hypoxia, 576–577

Apparent life-threatening events,
  amplitude-integrated EEG after,
  604–605

Asphyxia
  amplitude-integrated EEG in,
    603–605
  cerebral hemodynamic changes in, 718

Auditory system, neurodevelopment of, 700

Autoregulation, evaluation of, near-infrared
  spectroscopy in, 715–717

B

Bax protein, in hypercapnia, 585

Beer-Lambert law, in near-infrared
  spectroscopy, 708

Blood flow, cerebral
  in hypercapnia, 584
  measurement of, near-infrared
    spectroscopy in, 710
    autoregulation and, 715–717
    in preterm infant, 714–715

Blood pressure
  cerebral, measurement of, near-
    infrared spectroscopy in,
    autoregulation and, 715–717
  systemic, amplitude-integrated EEG
    and, 640–641

Blood sampling, umbilical cord, cerebral
  hemodynamic changes in, 717

Blood transfusions, cerebral hemodynamic
  changes in, 717

0095-5108/06/$ - see front matter © 2006 Elsevier Inc. All rights reserved.
doi:10.1016/S0095-5108(06)00071-6   *perinatology.theclinics.com*

Blood volume, cerebral, measurement of, near-infrared spectroscopy in, 709–710, 714–715

Brain
    injury of, **573–591**
        hypercapnia in, 584–587
        hypocapnia in, 577–584
        hypoxia in, 573–577
        mass spectrometry in, 738–740
    metabolism of, mass spectrometric monitoring of, 740–743
    plasticity of, sleep cycles and, 701–703

Brain monitoring
    added value in, 615–616
    data forms for, 615
    device operation for, 616
    for brain damage diagnosis, 616
    for ischemia, 613–614
    for research, 616–617
    for timely intervention, 613
    mass spectrometry in, **729–744**
    near-infrared spectroscopy in, **707–728**
    rationale for, **613–618**
    ST analysis studies in, 614–615

Brainstem auditory evoked potentials, in high-density EEG, 684

Bristol interactive course, for amplitude-integrated EEG, 669–672

C

Caffeine, cerebral oxygenation changes due to, 715

Calcium, in neurons
    hypocapnia-induced, 579–581
    hypoxia-induced, 573–575

cAMP-response element binding (CREB)
    in hypercapnia, 585–587
    in hypoxia, 574–575

Carbon dioxide
    abnormalities of. *See* Hypercapnia; Hypocapnia.
    vasoreactivity of, measurement of, near-infrared spectroscopy in, 711

Cardiac surgery
    cerebral hemodynamics during and after, 718–720
    seizures after, 655–658

Cardiopulmonary bypass, cerebral hemodynamics in, 718–720

Carnitine, mass spectrometric detection of, 730–731

Caspases, in hypoxia, 576–577

Cerebral function monitor. *See* Amplitude-integrated electroencephalography.

Cerebral monitoring. *See* Brain monitoring; Electroencephalography.

Cerebrospinal fluid aspiration, cerebral hemodynamic changes in, 717

Continuous electroencephalography. *See also* Amplitude-integrated electroencephalography.
    in seizures, 654–658
    in sleep monitoring, 703–705

Continuous wave near-infrared spectroscopy, 708

CREB (camp-response element binding)
    in hypercapnia, 585–587
    in hypoxia, 574–575

D

Deep hypothermic circulatory arrest, cerebral hemodynamics in, 718–720

Deoxyhemoglobin, measurement of, near-infrared spectroscopy in, 709–711
    in cardiac surgery, 719
    in fetus, 711–713

Diazepam, amplitude-integrated EEG changes due to, 639

Differential pathlength factor, in near-infrared spectroscopy, 708, 721

DNA fragmentation, in hypocapnia, 581–584

Documentation, of amplitude-integrated EEG, 673–676

Doppler ultrasound, for ischemia monitoring, 613–614

Doxapram, cerebral oxygenation changes due to, 715

E

EEG. *See* Electroencephalography.

Electrodes, for EEG, 672

Electroencephalography
    amplitude-integrated. *See* Amplitude-integrated electroencephalography.
    continuous. *See* Amplitude-integrated electroencephalography; Continuous electroencephalography.

high-density, **679–691**
in preterm infants. *See* Preterm infants.
in seizures. *See* Seizures.
in sleep, **693–706**
physiological basis for, **593–611**
staff training for, **667–677**

Electrographic neonatal seizure, definition
of, 654

Endogenous stimuli, in neurosensory
development, 698–700

Endotracheal suctioning, cerebral
hemodynamic changes in, 717

Evoked potentials, in high-density EEG,
680, 683–688
advantages of, 685
alternative analyses of, 685–686
brainstem auditory, 684
clinical application of, 684–685
visual, 683–688

Exogenous stimuli, in neurosensory
development, 698–700

F

Fetus, near-infrared spectroscopic
monitoring of, 711–713

Fick principle, for cerebral blood flow
calculation, 710

Flash visual-evoked potentials, in high-
density EEG, 683–685

FOS protein, in hypercapnia, 585–586

Free radicals, in hypoxia, 574, 576

Functional near-infrared spectroscopy,
720–721

G

Ganglion cells, retinal, development of, 698

Gavage feedings, cerebral hemodynamic
changes in, 717

Genomics, in mass spectrometry, 736–737

Gestational age
amplitude-integrated EEG and,
595–596, 602–603
high-density EEG and, 683–684

H

Heart surgery
cerebral hemodynamics during and
after, 718–720
seizures after, 655–658

Hemodynamics, evaluation of, near-
infrared spectroscopy in, 709–711, 715,
717–718

Hemoglobin, measurement of, near-infrared
spectroscopy in, 709–710
in cardiac surgery, 719
in fetus, 711–713

Hemorrhage, intraventricular
amplitude-integrated EEG in,
637–638
in hypercapnia, 584

High-density electroencephalography,
679–691
advantages of, 681–682
cap for, 681
in learning, 688–690
reference points in, 680
response to sensory novelty in, 688
safety of, 681
spontaneous measurement in, 680
synchrony in, 680–681, 686–688

Hypercapnia
amplitude-integrated EEG in, 641
brain injury in, 584–587

Hypocapnia
amplitude-integrated EEG in, 641
brain injury in, 577–584
calcium influx in, 579–581
DNA fragmentation in,
581–584
energy metabolism alterations in,
578–579

Hypoglycemia, electroencephalography in,
597, 641

Hypotension, amplitude-integrated EEG
and, 640–641

Hypoxia. *See also* Asphyxia.
brain injury in, 573–577
apoptosis in, 576–577
mass spectrometry in, 738–740
neuronal calcium influx in,
573–575

I

Ibuprofen, cerebral oxygenation changes
due to, 715

Indomethacin, cerebral oxygenation
changes due to, 715

Intraventricular hemorrhage
amplitude-integrated EEG in, 637–638
in hypercapnia, 584

Ischemia, cerebral, monitoring of, 613–614

L

Learning
  development of, 700–701
  EEG during, 688–690

M

Mass spectrometry, **729–744**
  clinical metabolomics and, 731–734
  for brain monitoring, 738–740
  for metabolic disease detection and
    monitoring, 730–737, 740–743
  for screening, 730–731
  future applications of, 730
  historical use of, 729–730
  principles of, 731
  samples for, 734

Mechanical ventilation, cerebral
  hemodynamic changes in, 717

Medium-chain acyl-CoA- dehydrogenase
  deficiency, mass spectrometry
  detection of, 732–736

Memory, development of, 700–701

Metabolic disorders, mass spectrometric
  detection of
  examples of, 731–734
  genomics in, 736–737
  history of, 730–731
  monitoring after, 740–743
  principles of, 731
  proteomics in, 736–737

Mismatch negativity, in high-density EEG,
  688

Monitoring, brain. See Brain monitoring;
  Electroencephalography.

Morphine, amplitude-integrated EEG
  changes due to, 639

N

Near-infrared spectroscopy, **707–728**
  artifacts in, 721–722
  clinical applications of, 711–715
  continuous wave, 708
  devices for, 708–709
  in cardiac surgery, 718–720
  in cerebral pressure monitoring,
    715–717
  in fetus, 711–713
  in functional activation studies,
    720–721
  in hemodynamic evaluation, 709–711,
    715, 717–718
  in interventions, 717–718
  in ischemia, 614

  in oxygenation measurement, 709–711
  in preterm infants, 713–715
  limitations of, 721–722
  phase-resolved, 709
  principles of, 707–708
  time-resolved, 709

Neurons, hypoxia-induced calcium in,
  573–575

Neurosensory development, sleep cycles in,
  698–700

Newborn Drug Development Initiative, 660

NIRS. See Near-infrared spectroscopy.

O

Octanoylcarnitine, mass spectrometric
  detection of, 732

Ocular dominance columns, 698

Oddball paradigm, in high-density EEG,
  688

Oxygen bolus technique, for cerebral blood
  flow calculation, 710

Oxygen free radicals, in hypoxia, 574, 576

Oxygen saturation, cerebral, measurement
  of, near-infrared spectroscopy in,
  710–711
  in fetus, 711–713

Oxyhemoglobin, measurement of, near-
  infrared spectroscopy in, 709–710
  in cardiac surgery, 719
  in fetus, 711–713
  in preterm infant, 714

P

Patent ductus arteriosus, amplitude-
  integrated EEG in, 641

Phase-resolved near-infrared spectroscopy,
  709

Phenobarbital
  amplitude-integrated EEG changes
    due to, 639
  for seizures, 658–660

Phenylalanine, mass spectrometric detection
  of, 732–733

Phenylketonuria, mass spectrometry in,
  732–733

Phenytoin, for seizures, 659

Plasticity, brain, sleep cycles and, 701–703

Presleep, 694–695

Preterm infants
    amplitude-integrated EEG in, **633–647**
        blood pressure effects on,
            640–641
        in carbon dioxide abnormalities,
            641
        in hypoglycemia, 641
        in intensive care, 641–642
        in intraventricular hemorrhage,
            637–638
        in patent ductus arteriosus, 641
        in sleep–wake cycle, 635–637
        in white matter injury, 637–638
        medication effects on, 638–640
        normal, 634–635
        practical aspects of, 642–643
    brain injury in
        causes of, 738–740
        in hypercapnia, 584–587
        in hypocapnia, 577–584
        in hypoxia, 573–577
        mass spectrometry in, 738–740
    brain monitoring in, rationale for,
        613–618
    near-infrared spectroscopy in, 713–715

Proteomics, in mass spectrometry, 736–737

Q

Quality control, of amplitude-integrated
    EEG, 675

R

Reporting, of amplitude-integrated EEG,
    673–676

Research, brain monitoring for, 616–617

Respiratory distress syndrome, near-
    infrared spectroscopy in, 716–717

Retina, neurodevelopment of, 698–700

S

Seizures, **649–665**
    electroencephalography in
        after heart surgery, 655–658
        alternative forms of, 660–662
        amplitude-integrated, 598–601,
            606–607, 625–627
        long-term, 654–658
        routine, 651–654
        subclinical, 650–651
            versus clinical events, 650–651
        treatment of, 658–660
        versus normal infant movements, 650

Sleep, **693–706**

continuous EEG monitoring in,
    703–705
development of, 693–696
    non-rapid eye movement,
        694–696
    rapid eye movement, 694–696
    species differences in, 694
historical studies of, 693–694
indeterminate (presleep), 694–695
non-rapid eye movement
    brain plasticity and, 702
    development of, 694–696
    in learning, 701
    in memory, 701
    in neurodevelopment, 697–703
    neurology of, 696–697
rapid eye movement
    brain plasticity and, 702–703
    development of, 694–696
    in learning, 701
    in memory, 701
    in neurodevelopment, 697–703
    neurology of, 696–697
stages of, 694

Sleep-wake cycle, EEG in, 606, 624,
    635–637

Sound stimuli, in neurosensory
    development, 700

Spectrometry, mass. *See* Mass spectrometry.

Spectroscopy, near-infrared. *See* Near-
    infrared spectroscopy.

ST analysis studies, 614–615

Stimuli, in neurosensory development,
    698–700

Suctioning, endotracheal, cerebral
    hemodynamic changes in, 717

Sufentanil, amplitude-integrated EEG
    changes due to, 639

Surfactant administration
    amplitude-integrated EEG in, 639
    cerebral hemodynamic changes in,
        717–718

Synchrony, in high-density EEG, 680–681,
    686–688

T

Thiopental, for seizures, 658

Time-resolved near-infrared spectroscopy,
    709

Topiramate, for seizures, 660

Training, for amplitude-integrated
electroencephalography, **667–677**
continuing, 669
electrode types and, 672
industry involvement in, 676–677
multiple channel, 672, 674
nationally recognized qualifications
for, 676
need for, 667–669
one-day interactive course for,
669–672
preliminary, 668–669
quality control in, 675
reporting of, 673–676
sequence for, 668

U

Umbilical cord blood sampling, cerebral
hemodynamic changes in, 717

V

Venous oxygen saturation, cerebral,
measurement of, near-infrared
spectroscopy in, 710–711

Ventilation, mechanical, cerebral
hemodynamic changes in, 717

Visual system, neurodevelopment of,
698–700

Visual-evoked potentials, in high-density
EEG, 683–688

W

White matter injury, amplitude-integrated
EEG in, 637–638

Moving?

Make sure your subscription moves with you!

To notify us of your new address, find your **Clinics Account Number** (located on your mailing label above your name), and contact customer service at:

E-mail: elspcs@elsevier.com

800-654-2452 (subscribers in the U.S. & Canada)
407-345-4000 (subscribers outside of the U.S. & Canada)

Fax number: 407-363-9661

Elsevier Periodicals Customer Service
6277 Sea Harbor Drive
Orlando, FL 32887-4800

*To ensure uninterrupted delivery of your subscription, please notify us at least 4 weeks in advance of move.